Practice-Based L
in Nursing, Health
Social Care

Practice-Based Learning in Nursing, Health and Social Care

Mentorship, Facilitation and Supervision

Ian Scott PhD, BSc, National Teaching Fellow (NTF)

Head of Academic Development and Practice
University of Worcester
UK

Jenny Spouse PhD, MSc Dip Nursing, Cert Ed, RNT, RCNT, RN, RM

Past Associate Dean for Practice Education
St Bartholomew School of Nursing and Midwifery
City University
London
UK

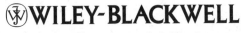

A John Wiley & Sons, Ltd., Publication

This edition first published 2013, © 2013 by John Wiley & Sons, Ltd.

Wiley-Blackwell is an imprint of John Wiley & Sons, formed by the merger of Wiley's global Scientific, Technical and Medical business with Blackwell Publishing.

Registered Office
John Wiley & Sons, Ltd, The Atrium, Southern Gate, Chichester, West Sussex, PO19 8SQ, UK

Editorial Offices
9600 Garsington Road, Oxford, OX4 2DQ, UK
The Atrium, Southern Gate, Chichester, West Sussex, PO19 8SQ, UK
111 River Street, Hoboken, NJ 07030-5774, USA

For details of our global editorial offices, for customer services and for information about how to apply for permission to reuse the copyright material in this book please see our website at www.wiley.com/wiley-blackwell.

Library of Congress Cataloging-in-Publication Data

Scott, Ian, 1964–
    Practice based learning in nursing, health and social care : mentorship, facilitation and supervision / Ian Scott, Jenny Spouse.
        p. ; cm.
    Includes bibliographical references and index.
    ISBN 978-0-470-65606-8 (pbk.)
    I. Spouse, Jenny.   II. Title.
    [DNLM: 1. Nursing–organization & administration–Case Reports.   2. Mentors–Case Reports.
3. Nurse's Role–Case Reports.   4. Nursing Theory–Case Reports.   5. Nursing, Supervisory–
Case Reports. WY 16.1]
    610.68–dc23

                                        2012040851

A catalogue record for this book is available from the British Library.

Wiley also publishes its books in a variety of electronic formats. Some content that appears in print may not be available in electronic books.

Cover image: iStock © Wojtek Piotrowski.
Cover design by Steve Thompson.

Set in 10/12.5pt Times by SPi Publisher Services, Pondicherry, India
Printed and bound in Malaysia by Vivar Printing Sdn Bhd

1   2013

Contents

About the authors

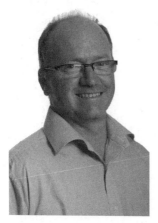

Dr Ian Scott

Ian is Associate Dean, Student Experience in the Faculty of Health and Life Science at Oxford Brookes University and has had a rich and diverse career within Higher Education. His first degree is in Applied Biology and he has a Ph.D. in Avian Ecology and Physiology. He has taught in a variety of Universities including Durham, De Montfort and City University, London. Whilst working for City University Ian developed a strong interest in; mentorship, research skill development and widening participation. He was awarded a National Teaching Fellowship in 2011. Ian lives in Worcestershire with his partner and two children. In his spare time he enjoys sailing and cycling, although not at the same time.

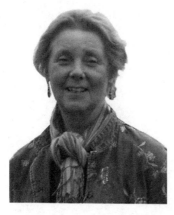

Dr Jenny Spouse

After spending several years nursing in Canada, Australia and Yemen, Jenny became a ward sister on a cardio-thoracic surgical ward at Barts Hospital, London. From this experience she developed a strong commitment to promoting professional education in the clinical setting. She became a clinical teacher and tutor for pre and post-registration nursing programmes, and subsequently Clinical Learning Environment Education officer at Oxford School of Nursing. After the transfer of Schools of Nursing and Midwifery into Higher Education, Jenny retained strong links with clinical practice, developing mentorship and assessment of practice programmes at Oxford, the Open University and St Bartholomew School of Nursing and Midwifery, where she was Associate Dean for Practice Education before retiring to become an educational consultant for the Open University. Jenny lives in Hampshire with a bouncy Labradoodle, which enjoys long countryside walks.

Chapter 1

Mentoring and supervision and other facilitative relationships

Ian Scott and Jenny Spouse

Introduction

In this chapter, we will be providing an overview to the text. We will discuss the origins of mentoring as a tool for personal development and its position within professional education from a macro- and micro-perspective. We will describe the increasingly important factors that are influencing the role, such as professional and national concerns, local and national policies. We will emphasise the critical importance of the person providing mentorship and who, in fulfilling their professional duty to protect the public, is both a gatekeeper to their profession and instrumental to the professional development of colleagues and visiting learners.

Throughout the chapter, we shall be exploring some of the vocabulary used across different professions to describe mentoring activities, and introducing and exploring some of the core concepts that are discussed in greater depth in later chapters.

This chapter includes the following:

- mentoring, coaching/supervision, the personal and professional implications of the role;
- what the different terminology means, for example, facilitator, mentor, supervisor, coach, sponsorship;
- introduction to the concepts of apprenticeship, communities of practice, sponsorship;
- the qualities of effective mentors to promote personal and professional development;
- the learner's perspective;
- learning and teaching.

Exploring the role of the practitioner teacher

Since ancient times, vocations have been learnt through practice by the aspirational learner working alongside an established practitioner. This way of learning has stood the test of time; it has been developed and expanded, and exists in many forms; and it is known by many names, but at its heart is one individual facilitating the learning of another through an individualised relationship. In the health professions, several terms are used to

Practice-Based Learning in Nursing, Health and Social Care: Mentorship, Facilitation and Supervision,
First Edition. Ian Scott and Jenny Spouse.
© 2013 John Wiley & Sons, Ltd. Published 2013 by John Wiley & Sons, Ltd.

identify such relations; it is common, for example, to find the terms mentor, supervisor and coach being used. In this book, will we commonly use the term 'mentor' or 'supervisor' to describe the person supervising and facilitating learning. We shall use the term 'learner' to describe a pre-qualification student as well as a qualified member of staff who is also a learner.

The term 'mentor' refers to the person who is helping the other person in the relationship learn, although quite often, the mentor will also be learning. If you have been asked or volunteered to help someone to learn in this way, then the world has honoured you, for helping someone to learn is a great gift to give, brings pleasure, will no doubt lead to your own personal and professional growth, and is in recognition of your own professional value and expertise. At some time during your journey in this role, you will want to develop and hone your skills as a mentor. Many people in this role not only have the responsibility of helping someone learn but also may have to make the decisions that will determine whether or not their learner can enter their profession. Working in this way means you have become a gatekeeper of the professional standards for your area of practice. This book is intended to help you to become that kind of gatekeeper to your profession. Through this text, we will explore the different aspects and skills of being a work-place facilitator in a health care setting, and as we do so we will introduce different ways of developing these skills. In writing this book, and through our own experiences, we are keenly aware that the process of facilitating is felt both ways by both learners and facilitators, and thus throughout the text, we have introduced the 'learner's perspective' often using real case studies from our experience and research.

Before we start getting down to the detail, it is worth spending some time exploring how the terms 'mentor', 'supervisor', 'facilitator' and 'coach' are used and in particular how they are used differently by different health professions. This is important because if we do not understand different professional terminology, discussions between professionals can become difficult. It will also help you to place your own workplace into the situations described in this book. Before we start this discussion, we want to emphasise that all of the terms used are equally correct. We just need to accept that the meaning placed on these terms varies a great deal across different professional groups.

Mentor

The first term we will look at is that of 'mentor'. The term 'mentor' is very widely recognised across organisations in the English-speaking world. It emerged largely in connection with large business organisations, where a 'mentor', normally someone successful at their business, would help another individual develop and succeed; the mentor's role was to offer advice and guidance to help the mentee form networks, and would also often act as a role model. The 'learning' aspect of the relationship was informal, as was often the formation of the relationship itself. Notice that the informal nature of this form of mentorship meant that the relationship developed between individuals that had 'attraction for each other'. For this reason, mentoring, although regarded as a route to success, was also considered to be a potential source of discrimination and potentially one of the reasons why certain groups within society (for example, women) are under-represented in the higher levels of top business.

Nevertheless, the role of the mentor as a significant person in an individual's development within a company or organisation was recognised, and this led to many organisations developing formal systems of mentoring. Probably the most common types of mentoring to be seen in organisations are those connected with the induction of individuals into the organisation. Here, a newly appointed member of staff is 'given' a mentor that will help the mentee 'find their feet' during the first few months of their new employment. Normally, after the induction period, the formal mentor/mentee relationship discontinues; it may, depending on the individuals, continue informally. In some organisations, there have been attempts to develop formal more prolonged periods of mentorship that attempt to mimic the initial form of mentorship that we described. In general, all the mentors described in the relationships above will have very little or no training for their role.

The last form of mentoring that occurs is that which has formal structures and rigid controls over who can mentor and how they are trained for the role. The mentoring role is closely tied to formal education programmes, and the mentor may well have a significant involvement in the summative assessment of their mentees. Many professions would call this form of relationship 'supervision' This form of mentorship can be seen in its most extreme form in relation to pre-registration education programmes for nurses midwives and social work within the within the United Kingdom, although in social work, the term 'mentor' is not used.

The term mentor itself, comes from ancient Greek mythology. Odysseus placed his son, Telemarchus, in the care of Mentor and Eumaeus; their relationship with Mentor was akin to that of teacher but also carer. An interesting twist in this tale is that Athena, a goddess of wisdom and war in Greek mythology, masqueraded as Mentor when she was trying to persuade him to follow her ideas and suggestions. You may want to consider which version of the mentor described above best fits with your experiences of being helped to develop your clinical practices.

Supervisor

The term 'supervisor' in the context of developmental relationships is harder to describe and find consensus for. The word supervision implies to oversee, and thus one thing we can say about these types of relationship is that they should be asymmetric; that is, the supervisor is normally in a more senior position to the supervisee. Such a term is used, for example, in universities in relation to learners being 'supervised' while they undertake projects. In many health care professions, however, the term 'supervisor' is used to describe a relationship whereby clinicians meet to discuss their practice with the purpose of improving it. Normally, however, one of the clinicians is more senior to the others. In nursing and midwifery practice, this form of supervision is often referred to as 'clinical supervision', but their activities are clearly much more focused on facilitating learning than on oversight. In some professions such as social work, the 'supervisor' is responsible for both providing opportunities for learning in practice settings and assessing whether the supervisee is fit to practise. Use of the term 'supervisor' in this way is synonymous with the term 'mentor' as used in the Nursing and Midwifery profession.

Interestingly, for the medical profession in the United Kingdom, 'supervised practice' is also the term used to describe the period of training and development that newly graduated medics undertake before becoming fully registered. Subjecting a qualified practitioner to supervision can also be applied by the General Medical Council as a sanction to a practitioner who has been found not to be fully competent.

Coach

The term 'coach' can be applied to a facilitative role or to describe a process and has become popular to describe a 'personal coach' who is used to assist their 'client' to make a lasting change in their behaviour. They do this by helping their client to establish their goals and the ways they will go about achieving these goals. A coach is intently focussed on helping their client 'find' their own way, rather than showing them the way. In general this kind of coach relationship with a client is less close than that of a 'mentor' and they are unlikely to be present and work alongside their client. In addition, unlike many mentor/supervisor relationships, the coach's career success does not tend to be linked to the success of their clients.

The exception to this would be the 'sports' coach. Use of the term 'coach' to describe a facilitative relationship is not commonly used within health care settings, but it is a term growing in popularity in the 'personal development' industry and so is likely to permeate the health care professions.

Obviously the terms 'mentor', 'coach' and 'supervisor' are used in different ways in differing context and have overlapping features. Unless your profession or your work place has adopted one of these terms and provided a clear definition, it is important that you qualify what you perceive your role to be, both for yourself and for the person you are working with. In this textbook, we will focus the discussion largely on the roles that relate to the descriptions of mentor and supervisor that we have given above. We will use the term 'coach' as a verb to describe some of the facilitative techniques used in 'coaching'.

Professional statutory regulatory organisations (PSROs)

Some PSROs regulate who can and cannot act as mentors/supervisors. For example, in the United Kingdom, the Nursing and Midwifery Council and the General Social Care Council have clear requirements of those wishing to act as a mentor or practice educator. These include successful completion of a prescribed training programme, the curriculum of which is largely dictated by the PSRO. Professional organisations normally require mentors/supervisors who are involved in the formal assessment of learners preparing for professional qualification (sometimes called neophyte – literally new growth) to be formally registered. The PSRO may also require further education and additional qualifications if a professional is taking on an extended role such as advanced prescribing. It is the case, however, in most countries that when ever a qualified professional is supervising another individual that could be deemed to be a 'learner', the qualified professional has the legal and ethical responsibility for the patients or clients in their care. Before taking on the role of a supervisor or mentor, it is a good idea to ensure that you are aware of the nature of this relationship and your own legal and professional responsibilities.

Apprenticeship and its relationship to mentorship and supervision

The term 'apprentice' seems to have emerged in the middle ages and is used in relation to the right of craftsmen to employ (at very low cost) boys that would provide labour in exchange for being trained into a particular craft or skill. Apprenticeships were highly prized, since, in the Middle Ages, becoming a craftsman or a professional was a route to a more secure future (just as it is today). Recognition as a craftsmen or 'professional' was through membership of a Guild. As the Guilds became successful and powerful, they sought to protect their reputation by imposing strict rules and regulations on their apprentices and guild members such as protecting the use of certain titles such as 'Stone Mason'. The Guilds regulated the terms of apprenticeships and controlled access to a wide range of professions. It is considered by some that the 'Guild' system led to the formation of Universities in the 12th century. Guilds covered a wide range of important economic activities, for example baking, brewing, weaving and carpentry. The authority of the Guilds was given to them by the monarch or the government of their respective nations. You can probably see in these Guilds similarities with modern professional regulatory organisations.

Interestingly, the Guilds system was largely abandoned by the 20th century. This is because they were seen as being highly protective, stifled innovation and were restrictive of free trade (Ogilvie 2004). Nevertheless many Guilds still have presence in modern times and are very influential in supporting charitable activities and promoting education.

An apprentice is thus someone who is learning a craft or profession through the process of watching and working alongside someone who is already fully capable with respect to that activity. The mode of learning would be best described as 'reproduction' learning or modelling. The apprentice would seek to mimic the actions of the master and thus acquire their skills. Modern forms of apprenticeship often include some form of formal study. Apprenticeships are often typified by apprentices having to practise and rehearse certain task over and over again, often irrespective of their actual level of competence (Singleton 1989).

Working and learning as apprenticeship

The nursing literature contains numerous accounts of nursing as an apprenticeship or sitting-by-nellie (Quinn 1981). There seems to be an implicit assumption that nursing learners were taught by an experienced artist or craftsperson at the bed side. The historical perspective of this is very different and more akin to that described by anthropologists of traditional craftsmen in apprenticeship (Maggs 1983). A number of studies from around the world demonstrate that apprentices are normally assigned to one master and work within a stable environment over a period of years. Throughout such arrangements, the master appears as a somewhat shadowy figure remote and impersonal, with apprentices relying on support from peers and experienced craftsmen (who may be masters to other learners) working within the workshop rather than with their own master (Coy 1989; Goody 1989; Singleton 1989). The organisation of such apprenticeship schemes was designed to enable learners to observe and later to participate in assigned and carefully structured tasks. Such tasks may be menial for a long time until the master believes the apprentice to be ready to undertake the next stage. Apprenticeship activities were carefully structured around repetitive activities that became increasingly sophisticated as apprentices demonstrated their worth. Theoretical information was obtained from talking to peers or another master. This model of learning relates very closely to the task-dominated wards of British general hospitals up until the end of the 20th century, and probably continues to exist in many health care settings. In these task-orientated settings, nursing learners were locked into the same type of progression as apprentices, by working through a scale of tasks. They had to practise these repetitively until they reached a more senior status within the organisation and could then be allowed to undertake a further series of more sophisticated tasks. Characteristic of this system is the most junior nurse being assigned the bed-pan rounds, cleaning the sluice and tidying the ward. After moving to the next ward or when another more junior learner arrived and s/he became more senior in the hierarchy, the learner is permitted to undertake more specialised procedures such as surgical dressings, management of intravenous infusions and drug administration. In the final year, learners are permitted to accompany doctors, to chaperone patients and to practise managing the ward. With few opportunities to observe another practitioner who is often hidden behind the screens, or engaged in more technical tasks, learners relied on gaining help from approachable peers. The role of the ward sister might have included some formal teaching, but this was only by chance and was often such an unfamiliar experience that the learner perhaps feared for the worse when s/he was summoned to the office for a tutorial.

In his discussion of common themes in adult industrial and professional apprenticeships, Graves argued that rites of passage created by obstructive and unhelpful behaviour of the 'masters,' were deliberately constructed to test learners' suitability for admission to the professionals' craft knowledge. These relationships were deliberately impersonal, competitive even combatory (Graves 1989: 51–64). Although his examples are concerned with men interacting using friendly but aggressive techniques that women may find threatening and destructive, there is evidence that nurses substituted such activities for their own with the same intent (Maggs 1983: 104). In order to survive, learners left the profession, adopted unacceptable behaviours such as erratic attendance or adopted the air of one who knew and thus became accepted by their seniors (Haas 1989: 102).

The ward sister as teacher in health care practice

Instrumental in fashioning the attitudes of nurses and teachers was a view that the 'art of nursing' could only be imparted through learners 'doing' and that their initiation into the art and science of their profession should take place at the bedside. It was also believed that this could be best achieved by delegating responsibility for learner teaching to one member of ward nursing staff (Lamond 1974: ix, 78). However, terms such as 'imparting values' and 'socialisation' are attached to these teaching activities. This suggests there was little perception that the actual nursing activities described as 'basic nursing care' required any teaching or guidance by clinical staff when a learner had arrived on the ward. Gott's observations indicated that ward teaching was associated with transmission of theoretical knowledge or techniques on which medical diagnosis and treatment, and thus the safety of the patient, may depend (Gott 1984: 68). Her observations were confirmed by several later studies, which demonstrated that supervision of learners was haphazard and that learners worked unsupervised for more than 75% of their clinical placement (Reid 1985; Melia 1987; Jacka and Lewin 1989). Earlier reports of the paucity of contact between learner and ward sister attributed the difficulty to the task-orientated management of nursing care as well as with high numbers of learners or other unqualified people staffing the wards (Nuffield Provincial Hospitals' Trust 1953). Two later studies investigating the nature of the clinical learning environment in general hospitals confirmed these findings and concluded that the nature of nursing management and staffing levels influenced opportunities for learning or teaching. This was hardly surprising if only one registered nurse (a ward sister or staff nurse) was on duty and responsible for supervising the care of 20 or more patients as well as the learners (Dodd 1973; Pearson 1978). There existed an assumption that learners' technical nursing knowledge would be acquired in the practical room of nursing schools and that they would arrive in practice as an essential part of the workforce, capable of fully undertaking the workload. Indeed, studies from this period implied that schools of nursing were failing to ensure learners were prepared for any incident that they may encounter in practice. The prime training task of ward staff was to teach learners the unusual and specialist technical skills. Such attitudes deny the complexity of everyday clinical practice and the uniqueness of delivering patient-centred nursing care. Such an interpretation explains Reid's findings that learners were more likely to receive supervision when undertaking a (high status) technical activity (Reid 1985: 73).

These research studies reflect nursing in the 1970s and perhaps earlier. It would be reasonable to believe that with better education and preparation of nurses, this research would be widely known, and changes will have taken place to improve the ward environment. Sadly, studies in the 1980s and 1990s demonstrated that learners continued to feel alienated by their clinical experiences and identified aspects of learning to nurse that would deter all but the committed (Hempstead 1988). Attrition (or 'wastage') from nursing, especially in the first year of training, has always been identified as problematic and expensive. MacGuire's extensive research of over 60 reports concerned with recruitment to, and withdrawal from, training from the period of 1940–1967 demonstrated that little had changed over the period reviewed and that learners left because of dissatisfaction with their working and living conditions (MacGuire 1970). Her conclusions were substantiated by later studies that specified reasons for learners feeling alienated from nursing. In particular, she found that they were stressed when left to encounter patients alone, particularly in the early part of their training when they lacked confidence in their interpersonal and practical abilities and knowledge of patients' needs (Birch 1975; Bradby 1990: 104; Seed 1995; Spouse 2003a, b). This unsatisfactory situation perhaps stems from the pervading assumption that providing care, more commonly described as 'basic nursing care', was routine and part of a common repertoire of human skills. Possibly this was true when the demography of society was different, sickness was more common, and most people were nursed at home. Nursing during these times recruited mature women who either were widowed or came from large families. Maggs cites Florence Nightingale as saying that the art of nursing was more than 'nursing one's own family as a loving daughter, wife or sister'. Perhaps she was implying that recruits were familiar with nurturing children or caring for the sick and for elderly relatives. Nurse training was concerned with transforming such elementary knowledge into artistry and a science through instruction and information on how to undertake specialised variations of techniques (Maggs 1983: 119). Magg's analysis of nursing and nurse education before the inception of the NHS contains much that is relevant to current experiences of learners learning, with a predominance of learning by trial and error (House 1977; Powell 1982; Mackay 1989; Bradby 1990: 136; Spouse 2003a, b). Inherent in the majority of research reports appears an assumption that with more and 'better' (formal) teaching, learners will learn. Nightingale's assertion that she cannot teach nurses but only point them in the direction of what to learn has perhaps been taken too much to heart. A consistent theme underlying all these reports is learners' dissatisfaction with their status as workers and the difficulties they experienced in receiving adequate support and supervision in their clinical placements. Contributing to this problem has been the conflicting interests of clinical practitioners charged with providing patient care and learner education. The over-dependence on learner labour as a prime source of care delivery with consequent insufficient qualified staff to provide supervision created significant tensions between idealised concepts of nursing and the bureaucratic needs of the hospitals (Gott 1984). Nurse teachers have been found wanting in meeting learners' learning needs in clinical practice, perhaps inevitably when considering the magnitude of their task.

More recent studies (Wisdom 2012) suggest that little has changed for the learner. This seems to be because of a reliance on care assistants, and later assistant practitioners, who have replaced the learner workforce with the introduction of the supernumerary status of learners with Project 2000 in 1989 and further in 1999 (UKCC Fitness for Practice). Yet evidence suggests that supervision by a knowledgeable practitioner, while undertaking practical care, is both valued and effective in developing learners' understanding and care (Alexander 1982; Spouse 1990; 1998; 2001; Wilson-Barnett et al. 1995).

Thus, the term apprenticeship has become synonymous with the notion of 'time served', that is, that the time served being an apprentice had significance and needed to be achieved. Thus, irrespective of the actual level of competence of an apprentice, learners would still need to complete their time. Apprentices often considered themselves cheap labour. Beyond the obvious (cheap labour) criticism of the apprenticeship approach, it is also attacked on learning and teaching grounds in that it supports the acquisition of the 'knowledge of action' and the uncritical reproduction of the model (master) which is a form of learning analogous to 'copying'. You may well question whether this is what is wanted in a caring profession. Probably not, and as a result, this form of apprenticeship model has been abandoned by the health care professions in favour of models that are more likely to lead to knowledge-driven, critically aware, innovative professionals.

The different forms of supervision that we have described are based on viewing learning in the workplace as learning that can be successful only when it is engaged with and is made possible through the support of a named learning facilitator.

You are not alone

As a mentor/supervisor, it is important that you recognise that it is unlikely that you are the only person acting in such a role within your organisation. You will have your own 'community of practice' where you can share your experiences with others in a similar role. Having supportive relationships with colleagues who understand the role is important to your own well-being. You need opportunities to discuss issues of interest and to learn from each other. It is likely that your organisation has its own network for meeting regularly. In addition, there are online networks and special-interest groups specially for health care professionals working as supervisors and mentors, for example, the coaching and mentoring network (http://www.coachingnetwork.org.uk/resourcecentre/whatarecoachingandmentoring.htm) and the network for mentors working in health settings in Scotland (http://www.flyingstart.scot.nhs.uk/mentor-area/mentor-networks.aspx), among many others. This process of forming a network like these is a first step to developing, or joining, a community of practice.

As discussed earlier in this chapter, the Guilds had many criticisms, but something that they certainly provided was the opportunity to create a common understanding, a place for shared learning, and a force to promote members and their actions (Ogilvie 2004). These aspects of Guilds can also be recognised as features of a community of practice. Lave and Wenger (1991) described a community of practice as made up of those 'participating in an activity system about which participants share understandings concerning what they are doing and what that means for their lives and for their communities'. As with any organisation, its success depends on each member using the same vocabulary and subscribing to the same values. This is socialisation, and if you are a new mentor, you may find it helpful to be sensitive to how your own language and attitudes are influenced by the group, as you will find that you are using similar techniques to socialise your mentee into your own workplace community of practice. Lave and Wenger's is not the only account and definition of a community of practice, and a good description and comparison of a range of ideas and thoughts on this subject have been provided by Cox (2005).

Why learning facilitators are important

The main way in which people learn is not through formal education in the classroom but informally through everyday activities within settings that are not designed for the purpose of learning. This type of 'everyday' learning is not structured and does not occur in discrete subjects; it is sometimes called experiential learning. Experiential learning, when it initially occurs, can seem rather chaotic, unordered and inefficient. The inefficiency is not hard to see; after all, this learning tends to be random, and we are not sure what learning opportunities may arise, and when. This form of learning, however, is extremely important because it is the principle way in which we develop our 'know-how' or tacit knowledge and develop skills. If we learn this way in our day-to-day lives naturally, you may ask 'Why do we need others to help us?' The role of those that facilitate learning, be they called mentors or supervisors, is to make this 'experiential learning' more ordered and more efficient. A good mentor, for instance, will remember that they need to help their mentee by finding suitable opportunities to learn. Where it is possible, they will create learning opportunities for them. They will also help their mentee to discover the learning that they have experienced through discussion and reflective practice. Another important action by mentors is to encourage their mentee to relate their new experiences to their existing knowledge.

Much learning that occurs is not obvious and stated; it is hidden. Indeed, the literature refers to it as the 'hidden curriculum'. A good example of this 'hidden curriculum' is the socialisation process, that is how professionals of one group 'learn' to talk and relate to those in another group or indeed how they learn the way a 'professional within their social group' dresses and behaves. In terms of this hidden curriculum, novices often learn by 'modelling' themselves on their mentors. Knowing that this form of learning is occurring is critical for a mentor to be aware of, because bad practice can be modelled as well as good if both the mentee and mentor are not critically aware of their practice.

Other roles and qualities of the mentor/supervisor

The roles described to the mentor in the literature are varied, and the qualities required often resemble a mixture that might be recognisable in saints or at least someone related to a saint. The roles have been placed into useful categories by several authors, although these categories are not necessarily the same. Box 1.1 illustrates Pawson's typology of roles or activities based on previous work by Kram (1985) and Eby (1997) that Pawson developed. He refers to these as mentoring mechanisms, and they are based on a wide range of mentoring situations. Box 1.1 lists descriptions of the ways that mentors can exert their influence, although not necessarily the way they should act.

In clinical settings, we would also want to add teaching, but Pawson's model certainly captures a significant number of the 'non-teaching'-related activities that a mentor/supervisor would be expected to undertake. Looking at these in turn:

Advocacy refers to the ways in which a mentor might work by:

- introducing their learner to colleagues and wider networks;
- finding opportunities for the mentee, and where necessary helping them to secure these opportunities;
- supporting (where appropriate) their mentee's decisions and generally using their influence within the organisation to enhance the development of their mentee.

Coaching activity, for Pawson (2004), is about 'encouraging, pushing and coaxing their protégés into practical gains, skills and qualifications' (Pawson 2004: 7). We would add that as 'coach', the mentor works by helping the mentee to see what their strengths are and to orientate their goals; for the coach mentor, attainment of measurable goals is very important.

When a mentor is '*Direction setting*', they are offering advice, particularly where difficult decisions are being taken.

As an *emotional resource*, the mentor is acting as confidant and friend.

Box 1.1   Pawson's mentoring mechanisms (Source: Pawson 2004).

Advocacy (positional resources)
Coaching (aptitudinal resources)
Direction setting (cognitive resources)
Affective contacts (emotional resources)

Pawson (2004)

In clinical situations where the mentor/supervisor may also be an assessor and guardian of patients' and clients' safety, some of the 'mechanisms of mentoring' will not work, or certainly can create tensions. It is difficult to see, for example, how a supervisor can be both a formal assessor and a confidant and maintain objectivity in relation to the assessment.

Point to ponder:
Which of Pawson's categories do you think coincides with your own experiences of mentoring to date?

Expressed in more pragmatic terms, McKimm et al. (2007) produced the following list (Table 1.1) of activities that mentors were likely to undertake in the clinical setting; we have removed references to those activities that relate directly to the role of teacher.

Fortunately, the list compiled by McKimm et al. (2007) and that of categories provided by Pawson (2004) have considerable degree of overlap. McKimm et al.'s list also has considerable overlap with the activities of mentors described by Hay (1995) and Darling (1984). Their list of qualities also based around the ideas of Hay and Darling, required of mentors is a bit scarier (Table 1.2).

You have probably concluded that this list is not exhaustive, and some qualities are more important than others. To possess all these qualities and to be able to use them all the time would be a great achievement, and probably few of us would be able to succeed. It is, however, worthwhile being aware of these qualities and activities described in Tables 1.1 and 1.2, because to be a successful mentor or supervisor, you will need to use many of them.

Table 1.1   Activities of mentors adapted from those described by McKimm et al. (2007).

Translator and decoder, for example, of organisational culture and values	Critic
Confidante counsellor	Energiser
Interpreter	Guide
Motivator	Sounding board
Time manager	Taskmaster
Facilitator	Devil's advocate
Planner	Sponsor
Coach	Protector
Problem-solver	Process consultant
Friend	Role model
Adviser	Target setter
Diagnostician	

Points to ponder:
Look at this table, and think about the extent to which you have used these activities in the mentoring or supervision that you have done thus far. Give yourself a score from 1 to 5 (5 being the most).
Are there any additional activities you could add to the list?

McKimm (2007).

Table 1.2   Qualities of mentors adapted from those described by McKimm et al. (2007).

Good interpersonal skills	Good interpersonal skills · objectivity
Objectivity	Role model
Role model	Flexibility
Flexibility	Command peer respect
Peer respect	Demonstrable competence
Demonstrable competence	Reflective practitioner
Reflective	Empathy
Non-threatening attitude	Advocacy
Facilitator of learning	Sincerity
Allowing the development of independence	Sincerity
Open-mindedness	Warmth
Approachability	Commitment
Self-confidence and self-awareness	Understanding
·	Aptitude for the role

Points to ponder:
Look at the table, and think about the extent to which you have used these qualities in any mentoring or supervision you have done so far. Give yourself a score between 1 and 5 (5 being the most).
Can you think of any other qualities to add to this list?
Now ask a friend to rate you on the same scale of 1–5.
How closely does your own score match those given to you by your friend?

McKimm (2007).

What about the learner perspective?

It is worth asking the question, where did the information in Tables 1.1 and 1. 2 come from? Was it just the authors' thoughts? Are they the thoughts of those facilitating learning or learners? The answer is probably a mix of all three, although within the literature, there is some concern that the learner's voice is often missed. In addition, the research cited above does not capture any real idea of what are learners' top priorities in relation to the capabilities and qualities of their facilitator. Gray and Smith (2000) interviewed nursing learners and asked how they would 'be' if they were mentors. These learners reported that if they were mentors, they would:

- form a relaxed relationship with their learner;
- support the learner, rather than breathe down their neck;
- encourage and allow involvement and participation in patient care, rather than just observation;
- show confidence in the learner's abilities and trust them to do things unsupervised;
- take time every day to let the learner do or observe something and not assume that because they were in a certain term, they would have already seen or performed it;
- regardless of the learner's stage, have an initial discussion preferably on the first day, to determine what the learner's present abilities were and their intended learning outcomes (a term used to describe what will be learnt at the end of a period of learning) for the placement;
- ascertain what the learner required as an individual to meet the desired learning outcomes;

- clarify ground on both sides and discuss the opportunities available to meet desired learning outcomes;
- remember the learner if there was anything interesting happening in the clinical area;
- allow the learner some independence by giving more guidance at the beginning of the placement; then, they would stand back and let the learner show initiative and self-motivation;
- make arrangements with other members of staff to 'look out for them' if they were going to be off duty when the learner was on duty, rather than have the learner feel abandoned;
- think carefully about the duty rota in terms of arranging shifts to allow learner and mentor to work together at some point each week.

While these views from nurse learners, mostly on placement with hospital wards, seem to be informed by negative experiences, they do accord with the general literature on mentoring and supervision, and with others who have researched the experience of this group of learners (e.g., Spouse 1996). Gray and Smith's study is also particularly interesting, because it highlights the value mentees place on their mentors' being realistic, enthusiastic and positively disposed towards their profession. Their work suggests that it is important to learners that mentors hold their own profession in high regard and believe it to be worthwhile. It also suggests that 'putting a profession or a role down' should be something to avoid.

Attributes and knowledge for the learning and teaching role

So far, we have argued that the main role of the mentor is to facilitate learning and therefore to make the process of experiential learning more efficient. To do this in addition to those attributes described in Tables 1.1 and 1.2, it is important for you to have a good understanding of how to facilitate learning and to appreciate the personal attributes that are more likely to ensure a supportive, mutually beneficial relationship.

The terms 'learning' and 'teaching' is worth exploring. They are used widely by educationalists to encapsulate purposeful activities and actions (teaching) that lead to learning. It stands to reason that someone who is facilitating another's learning will need to know about 'learning' and the processes that are effective in helping others to achieve this learning.

The term 'learning' is harder to define than teaching, and indeed the definitions vary depending on the source that you are using. In addition, it has also been recognised for some time that there are different types of learning and knowledge. Simple definitions of learning include:

1   *Learning concerns the acquisition or modification of knowledge, skills and behaviours.* Like most simple definitions of complex things, it hides more than it actually reveals! What, for example, is meant by knowledge, and does it include knowing how to do things with 'knowledge'? Ormrod (1999) gives two definitions
2   *Learning is a permanent change in behaviour*

3   *Learning is a relatively permanent change in mental associations due to experience.*
You may note that in this definition, sitting in a class room listening to someone also
counts as experience.

Definition 1 describes a number of situations in which learning can take place, covering
practice as well as academic study, but this does not necessarily cover all forms of learning
experiences. Ormond's two definitions of learning require evidence that something has
changed. Thus, in definition (2), reading a book on history may result in you acquiring
new facts and understanding, but under this definition, it is not learning. Definition (3) has
the most application, as it does not muddle us by talking about different types of things
that may be learnt. It describes learning as making 'new' mental associations.

It could be argued that many of the processes that support learning are probably known
intuitively; after all, we imagine that most parents seem instinctively to know how to help
their offspring learn skills of survival in modern society. Other types of learning, however,
the types that we would equate with the knowledge and skills required to be a health care
professional, require more than this instinctive ability, and indeed if we look around, we
will know that some people are better at helping others acquire practical or technical
knowledge than others.

Point to ponder:
Think about someone whom you admire as a good teacher.

- What attributes do they have that makes them memorable?
- Do you think you might have adopted any of their attributes when facilitating learning
  in others?
- Which of your attributes might others adopt in their own work?

The workplace and learning

The exact nature of learning opportunities depends upon each individual learner and how
they learn. The learning itself takes place in what is called a placement, which may or may
not have an environment that promotes learning (the learning environment). The concept
of a learning environment describes not only the setting where learning takes place but the
quality of the professional activities, the abilities of the resident and visiting practitioners,
and their ability to provide learning opportunities. Building a series of opportunities, for
a particular learner, in a particular environment, is sometimes referred to as a learning
strategy. It is sometimes easy to lose sight of how learning in the workplace happens. You
may find a model created by Beard and Wilson (2002; 2006) useful. They have identified
six core aspects of learning. The six core aspects they identify are:

- belonging;
- doing;
- sensing;
- feeling;
- thinking;
- being.

Belonging is the notion that learning depends on the learning feeling that they are part of a community and the setting. It includes notions of place, culture and local socio-political context, and can be summed up in the term used earlier: the 'learning environment'.

Doing is the representation of the 'Learning Activities'; these are the things that the learner does that give rise to learning.

Sensing concerns how information is received internally for processing, by the learner; this area is particularly complex, since people vary in their preferred way to receive information.

Feeling embodies the emotions that are involved in learning, which can be very profound when learning in clinical settings and greatly influence what, how and the quality of our learning; in some books, this may be referred to as the affective domain of learning. It includes those things that influence attitudes, motivation and the valuing placed on what is being learnt.

Thinking or cognition refers to those mental activities that help us to internalise knowledge and to gain understanding; it includes processes such as comprehending, applying knowledge to new problems, analysing, synthesising, evaluating and reflecting.

Being is the act of change in a person being caused and the learning occurring. The act of learning influences the other core aspects. Beard and Wilson (2002; 2006) view these aspects as existing in a dynamic change, each interlinked but able to have different levels of prominence depending on the learner and their situation.

For learning to be successful, it is important for the learner and supervisor/mentor to determine and agree the professional needs, or goals, of the learner. This process is always based on some form of assessment. It is often taking place continuously although as a sub-conscious activity. When you are facilitating formal 'accredited' learning, this identification of needs is often based on a series of learning outcomes. Indeed, very often learners come from their Adult Education Institution armed with a set of predetermined learning outcomes.

Learning outcomes are statements of what should be achieved following engagement with a range of learning opportunities. Writing learning outcomes that are comprehensible and usable is always a challenging activity; in fact they are a complex concept masquerading as a simple one (Scott 2011).

Learning opportunities are the activities that learners need to engage in, and will include things such as: developing an understanding of different health care pathways in the community and a range of institutions; understanding the work of a wide range of associated health care professionals; participating in managing and delivering a wide range of health care activities; dialogue with clients, carers and colleagues; joining and functioning effectively within a health care team; developing their evidence-based knowledge; and personal development.

At the end of the period of learning, it is always important to evaluate whether or not your facilitation strategy was successful. In other words, to what extent the desired learning outcomes have been achieved, or whether different learning outcomes from those intended have also been achieved. This process of evaluation, by necessity, involves some form of assessment; in many circumstances, the evaluation and assessment will and should be ongoing. Documenting your findings from your assessment is a vital part of the mentor role, as it provides your learner with evidence of what they have achieved and what is outstanding. In the rare situation where your learner's standard of performance is unsatisfactory, your documented records of your assessments, the actions and the outcomes provide evidence that is vital for making fair and proper decisions that could save someone's life.

Summary

From what you have read in this chapter, you can appreciate that mentorship or supervision of novices has a long and important history. Throughout this book, we will consider factors that contribute to learning in practice settings, take you through the learning process from the perspective of both the learner and the mentor, examine ways in which facilitation skills can be developed, and provide information, ideas and activities to inform your own practice as a supervisor and as a professional.

Because we believe that learning is more effective when the reader is actively engaged, in the text we have included some vignettes and snapshots that illustrate how our main points could be applied to everyday professional practice. We have also included some questions (Points to Ponder and Socratic Questions) that we think will help you to learn, and we hope you will answer them before progressing to the next section of the book.

We have written this text so that each of the main chapters can be read in isolation from the others, although of course we would prefer you to read the whole text. At the end of reading the book, we are certain you will have a better understanding of how to facilitate the learning of other individuals in your workplace and be more effective in your role as a facilitator. Enjoy!

Chapter 2

Personal and professional aspects of supervising others

Jenny Spouse

Introduction

Most practitioners become mentors of learners by default. Some describe it as 'Baggins' turn'. This is a pity, as mentoring a learner can be an enriching as well as a challenging experience. Many practitioners feel that they benefit from the relationship, saying that it helps to keep them up to date as well as 'keeping them on their toes'. The greatest challenge is being able to fit 'it' all in. The combination of a full workload with the addition of supporting one or more pre-registration course learners as well as other colleagues who are also learning on the job is a tall order. This chapter aims to help you to develop strategies to address such challenges. It has six sections that address a different aspect of the mentoring role. Some of the strategies are designed to help you to avoid difficulties and others to help you in your everyday practice. The first sections are concerned with your professional obligations, and then we go on to exploring strategies to maximise the benefits for your learner, your patients/clients and your colleagues as well as yourself.

This chapter includes the following:

- creating a learning partnership, being a newcomer, establishing the relationship;
- professional boundaries and responsibilities, including duty of care, dealing with unsatisfactory conduct; educational responsibility and professional accountability;
- the learner's perspective on supportive relationships;
- models of mentoring/supervision;
- approaches to mentoring;
- emotional labour and mentoring.

Creating a learning partnership: ways in which relationships between learner and facilitator enhance learning

Being a newcomer

You may have memories of being a newcomer in unfamiliar surroundings. Most of us have had a change of schooling that meant existing friendships changed, and new ones

Practice-Based Learning in Nursing, Health and Social Care: Mentorship, Facilitation and Supervision, First Edition. Ian Scott and Jenny Spouse.
© 2013 John Wiley & Sons, Ltd. Published 2013 by John Wiley & Sons, Ltd.

had to be developed. Even walking into an unfamiliar town, street or shop can lead to some unease until we know our way around and are familiar with the street signs. If we are in an unfamiliar country, our unease usually remains until we know enough of the local customs and language to be understood and to regain some self-confidence. Many people are unwilling to venture to a country where a different language is used for fear of feeling inadequate in some way. And yet learners undergoing a professional programme are often exposed to as many as six to 12 very different environments during their pre-registration programme. Each time they are allocated to an unfamiliar clinical placement, they have to establish relationships with the staff, learn about the local customs and routines, the rules and requirements as well as those rules and requirements that are hidden. Often, the everyday language of the clinical setting includes words that are unfamiliar and hold specific meanings that as a newcomer the learner has to learn. During the first year and particularly first placement experience, learners often find such encounters completely disabling – a sense that never disappears entirely throughout their programme.

It is not uncommon for many learners to be greeted with surprise by on-duty staff when they first appear on their placement and told that they were not expected. 'No one told us you were coming' is a familiar cry that most learners will have heard at one time or another. Not quite the welcome an enthusiastic junior learner expects, and always indefensible irrespective of the truth of the matter. Inevitably, there is a responsibility on the learner to find out as much about the placement as they can before they start. With more placement areas having access to intranet resources, clinicians with an educational responsibility often post information about their clinical speciality and the key figures within the setting. This helps newcomers to prepare for their placement as well as to familiarise themselves with the everyday professional vocabulary of the setting. Making a preliminary visit to their new placement for many, quite impoverished learners may not be possible if the university is several miles from their home and even further from their placement. But if early contact can be initiated by email, text or Skype, both learner and their mentor can begin to establish a working relationship. Various studies have identified the following factors that influence the success or otherwise of newcomers arriving in a new working environment.

Being welcomed to an unfamiliar setting, and so by definition a potentially hostile environment, by a key member of the staff is one of the most important aspects of ensuring the successful progress of the learner. Research by Nicholson (1987) found that people who were not encouraged to join the working community or group, or who were not given a social identity, soon left the community. Another study by Fuhrer (1993) demonstrated that newcomers, or people entering a potentially hostile social setting inevitably sought somewhere out of the way and where they hoped they would not be noticed. Newly arrived learners who are not welcomed and looked after often feel like running away (see research by Spouse 1998). This could explain why some learners have high levels of sickness and absence when on placement or why some give the impression of being reluctant to engage in the social situation of the placement. As a result, the practitioners of the community are more likely to reject the newcomer even further and thus shut them out completely to their own detriment as well as to the learner.

Writers on causes of oppression identified four key social factors that lead to humans feeling oppressed or disempowered (Carr & Kemmis 1986):

- *The concrete social experience* – whether the newcomer is welcomed into the community or is ignored.
- *Personification of participants* – the extent to which the person is encouraged to engage in the everyday activities of the community and to have a recognised role.
- *Analysis of their experience* – how the individual perceives and interprets their experience against their existing knowledge and beliefs. So, a newcomer who has had an unwelcoming experience previously is likely to be more anxious than one who has only encountered positive experiences.
- *Contextual operating mechanisms* – these may be related to the policies of the clinical organisation such as whether learners are allowed to take their meal breaks or to participate in social activities with the staff. By contrast, it could be related to what is happening in the learner's personal life, whether s/he has financial worries or housing problems that are a distraction.

You are probably familiar with the work of Abraham Maslow (1970), whose research indicated that physical and social needs had to be met before effective intellectual activities such as learning can take place. This can perhaps explain the behaviour of those who are left out in the 'cold' by their new peers. When free from a constant fear of rejection, newcomers and learners can concentrate on learning and engaging productively within the social setting. It is possible that the physical and emotional relaxation that follows acceptance within a social group enables people to be aware of what is taking place around them and to learn.

Establishing the relationship

The most important factor that influences the success or failure of a newcomer is the extent to which they are supported by a key member of the community. Research by two educational anthropologists studying learning in practical settings across different cultures called such a person a 'sponsor' (Lave & Wenger 1991). In her research into how nursing learners developed their professional knowledge, Spouse (2003a, b) found that without the support of a sponsor, learners felt isolated and invisible while at the same time feeling unbearably self-conscious. The sponsor did not need to be their personal mentor, but it did need to be someone who took responsibility for their well-being and professional development in that setting and who had the respect of the other members of the social group. Spouse (2003a, b) described this sponsorship by the learner's mentor as 'befriending' and argued that learning was more effective, and learners were then able to contribute substantially to the team as a whole when they were befriended by their mentor. She describes this as a relationship that is based on mutual trust and respect, that provides the learner with a 'secure base' (Bowlby 1988) and that facilitates learning opportunities. Jones (2010) supports this argument and draws on research from New Zealand (Vallint and Neville 2006) that also illustrates the importance of learners feeling part of the clinical team. Other researchers describe this as 'belongingness' (Levett-Jones et al. 2007) and argue that it is the keystone to learners' success in developing the necessary professional skills.

Developing such a trusting relationship takes dedicated time and a willingness to be open to each other. It provides an opportunity for mentor and mentee to learn about each other. If, as a mentor, you have a sense of your learners' personal and educational background, then you are more able to tailor their learning experiences. If you know that your learner is a single mother with a nursery-aged child living in rented accommodation, then you are likely to have a different perspective than if you see her as fresh out of school and living in university halls.

Each learner has a different pattern of placement experiences, and thus their technical or professional knowledge is going to be different. It is going to be even more different if their previous mentors have been too pre-occupied with their clinical activities to provide educational supervision. Learners who have the latter experience of mentoring tend to be severely disadvantaged and struggle to keep up with their peers. Even though learners preparing on different programmes now carry a professional portfolio or a passport record of their clinical experiences, it does not necessarily provide an accurate account of their progress. Expectations may vary from placement to placement, as might attitudes to learners.

By engaging in a Befriending activity, you are providing your learner with what Bowlby (1988) described as a 'secure base'. As a result, learners feel 'freed up' to be more authentic or to be themselves and thus to relax and to be open to learning as well as to correction. As a result, their confidence grows, and they are more able to take on responsibility for their own learning. They can also make greater use of learning opportunities and to learn from others. Establishing a mutually respectful and trusting relationship with your learner offers you some security to know that your learner will discuss any anxieties they have and to be forthcoming if they feel they have made a mistake. For the learner, it can reduce the sense of being a burden on their mentor and increase their sense of being a (junior) partner in care delivery and thus motivates them to be willing and to engage fully – surely a win–win relationship.

Professional boundaries including duty of care, professional accountability and educational responsibility

Duty of care

As a registered practitioner, you have a duty of care towards your clients or patients, who are vulnerable to any form of abuse. Abuse may be caused by ignorance as well as by malpractice (including negligence) or omission of care. This is a heavy responsibility for a registered practitioner, when already burdened by the responsibilities for a busy clinical work load while supervising colleagues and learners with a range of personal and professional backgrounds. Being conscious of the boundaries of your own responsibilities provides a basis for your decision-making regarding delegation of activities. It also helps you to make explicit the boundaries of your colleagues' (peers, learners) responsibilities and for what they are accountable. Knowing the abilities and limitations of your colleagues' professional practice means you are able to delegate effectively and safely. It also makes it more likely that your patients/clients will receive satisfactory standards of care.

As a mentor and a registered professional practitioner, you are bound by your professional Code of Conduct. This requires you to demonstrate competence at all times and to maintain your fitness to practise. This does not require you to be all-knowing, but to be aware of your limitations and to take the necessary actions to address them. The Code also requires you to ensure that all people are treated fairly and equally according to their religious beliefs and irrespective of their race or gender. This means that anyone for whom you are responsible, irrespective of whether you are the primary or the secondary person, are dependent upon your own professional standards and judgement. So, if you delegate tasks to a colleague or to a learner, you are obliged by the Code of Professional Conduct to satisfy yourself that the practitioner is competent and capable of delivering the appropriate care. This can be achieved only by direct supervision and observation of their practice. You also need to ensure that their workload does not hamper their capability to deliver a high standard of care. As a registered practitioner responsible for the care of a group of patients you need to create an environment of trust where colleagues who are working with you can feel confident to acknowledge their limitations and to receive continuing education as needed. This is a demanding requirement from your professional regulatory body. Their concern is to protect the public and to ensure the continued high standard of the profession. This is a particularly demanding requirement when health and social care providers responding to government funding cuts reduce the numbers of qualified professional practitioners and increase the number of untrained ancillary staff, often leaving unqualified staff to support learners.

Responding to unsatisfactory practice

Taking action following evidence of unsatisfactory practice is a crucial part of fulfilling your duty of care. This action includes correcting the person whose practice is unsatisfactory, notifying the appropriate authorities, documenting the unsatisfactory practice and the actions taken to address the problem. Depending upon the nature of the unsatisfactory practice, remedial support is normally required, and the person is not permitted to engage in the same level of unsupervised activity until they have demonstrated a consistent and satisfactory level of practice.

If you receive evidence of poor-quality practice that requires immediate suspension of the practitioner pending an investigation, then as the practitioner with overall responsibility for your client or patient's care, you need to obtain support from your immediate manager as a matter of urgency. You also need to document the incident clearly and precisely as soon as possible. This documentation must include the date and time of the incident, the names of the persons involved, the precise nature of the incident and your signature. Your organisation will have a policy that explains exactly what needs to be done and by whom.

This principle applies whether it is a member of staff or a visiting learner. Fortunately, such incidents are relatively rare, but the principle of taking such prompt action is an essential part of your duty of care towards the vulnerable, both in the present and in the future (Vignette 2.1).

Vignette 2.1   Jose's dilemma

Jose is working with her first learner as the primary mentor, a second-year nursing student, Jack. They have worked together on the same shifts for the past two weeks. During this time, Jose has had some reservations about Jack and his professional conduct but not had any concrete evidence to confirm her concerns. This morning, after having discussed their workload and agreed how to share it, Jack is caring for four high-dependency residents. After giving out the medications, Jose leaves Jack with the agreed care plan and asks him to come and find her if he needs any help. At 9.45 am, Jose goes in to see the residents and see how Jack has been getting on. She is disconcerted to find that only one resident has been helped to sit by her bed, and the others are still in bed. She is even more concerned to find that they have been waiting for Jack to take them to the toilet for the past 90 min, with inevitable consequences. Jack is nowhere to be seen and does not appear to be on site. Jose alerts her manager and the security staff, who search the grounds with no success. At 11.30 am, Jack is seen walking down the corridor. His allocated residents have not seen him all morning, and Jose has been looking after them in Jack's absence. Jose finds Jack and suggests they go into the office for a talk.

Points to ponder:

What do you think Jose may have in mind to say to Jack?
What do you think Jose's responsibilities are towards her residents and towards Jack?
What actions do you think Jose needs to take regarding Jack's behaviour?
Who do you think Jose should inform regarding Jack's behaviour?

At first glance, Jack's behaviour was a serious breech of his duty of care towards these people. Whatever reasons he had for leaving his clients, he was wrong to leave them without telling Jose what he was doing and why. Jose now has the difficult task of managing the situation and minimising any further harm to the people under her care now and in the future. A critical aspect of her management and educational responsibilities is to ensure that the incident is accurately documented according to the organisation's procedures, as well as to document the incident in Jack's records. Jack's university may have some guidelines or a procedure for mentors to use, and this will probably include notifying the professional person responsible for learners on placement in the residential homes as well as Jack's personal tutor. Jack's behaviour may lead to him being suspended from his programme pending an investigation by the university. The team of investigators (normally an academic and a placement representative) will need a well-documented account of the incident to help them come to a decision that is fair and appropriate. If as for example in Jack's case (Vignette 2.2) this is not the first time that his conduct has been inappropriate, it is likely that he will face dismissal from his programme. It is probable that he will appeal, and his appeal will be supported by his student union and will be heard by a university tribunal. Having documented evidence of the incident and the support provided enables the tribunal to make the most appropriate decision. Vignette 2.2 is an illustration of what Jose might have written in her report of the incident.

Vignette 2.2   Documenting Jack's behaviour

Incident on date: XXX at time 9.45 am–11.30 am

Jack Dunse (second-year nursing student) had been allocated to look after five medium-dependency residents, with the distant supervision of his mentor (Jose Makepeace). At the beginning of the shift, Jack and I discussed the care plans for each patient along with his plans for managing the morning's work. After administration of medications at 9 am, Jack assured me that he was confident to deliver the agreed plan. I then left Jack to attend to the remaining patients, having satisfied myself that Jack was capable of delivering the care prescribed according to the agreed management plan.

At 9.45 am, I went to see how he was getting on and discovered that the residents had not seen him since I had left him at 9 am. Searching the unit, Jack was nowhere to be found. I contacted the manager of the unit and informed her of the situation. She contacted security and asked them to search the building and the grounds for Jack, but he was not to be found on the site. At 11.30, Jack appeared, as if nothing had happened and, when asked where he had been, was unable to give a satisfactory answer. He acknowledged that he had not informed anyone that he was leaving the Unit and the site.

A meeting was convened between Jack, Jose Makepeace and the Nursing manager of the home at 12md. Jack was asked to give an explanation for his absence. He replied that he had gone down to the shops to buy some cigarettes for one of the residents, Mr Caine. He acknowledged that he had not informed anyone of what or where he was going. He argued that as he was a supernumerary student, he felt it did not matter if he left the unit.

The Nursing Manager explained to Jack that as he had accepted responsibility for a group of patients and that he had agreed to use the management plan for the morning's work, his absence without notifying his supervisor was unprofessional and had placed his patients at risk. She reminded him that although he was classified as a supernumerary student, it did not allow him to abdicate his agreed responsibilities. His behaviour was serious and in breach of his Professional Code of Conduct. She explained that she would be contacting his personal tutor and would be writing a report of the incident on behalf of the university. She further explained that he may have to attend a disciplinary hearing and that if he repeated the behaviour he would no longer be accepted on the placement.

The report was subsequently dated and signed by Jack as a true record of the event and countersigned by Jose and the Nursing Manager.

Points to ponder:

How do you think Jack may be feeling as he signs this report?
Why do you think it is important that Jose and the Nursing manager document the incident?
What may be the consequences of documenting the incident for: (1) Jack? (2) Jose and her Nursing manager?
Reading through this report, do you have a clear understanding of the event?
If Jack does face a disciplinary hearing, perhaps two months later, do you think the panel members will appreciate the seriousness of Jack's actions from this information?
What do you think should happen if Jack repeats his actions?
How might your own organisation deal with such an incident?

It is possible that this is not the first time for Jack to have behaved in this way. His argument of being a supernumerary student and thus not included in the workforce numbers seems quite plausible, superficially. However, by accepting responsibility for a group of the residents, he has a duty of care towards them and to the organisation, and thus is not a free agent. If he had behaved in this way on a different placement, why does he still feel that his actions were quite legitimate? Could it be that no one appeared to take his behaviour seriously enough to document the incident? Having the kind of detailed documentary evidence in Vignette 2.2 enables Jack's personal tutor, as well as the placement manager, to deal with it in an effective way. If, for example, this is the second or third time that Jack had been told that this behaviour was unprofessional, and his tutor has documentary evidence, then it is possible to suspend Jack from his studies pending a disciplinary hearing and possible dismissal from his course. Without such evidence, other than perhaps a note in his placement report alluding to his behaviour, then there is little that can be done, and it is probable that Jack will continue to feel that his behaviour is acceptable.

There is a large amount of evidence from research (Duffy 2003) that learners who are allowed to continue with unsatisfactory practice struggle to improve. They are invariably let down by their mentors who are reluctant to fail them, thus releasing them as a registered practitioner onto an unsuspecting clinical team and, more importantly, to the vulnerable patient. If the learner's needs had been respected and their mistakes used as learning opportunities, it is possible that they would have had an opportunity to develop appropriately. When a learner demonstrates poor practice, attitudinal or technical, such events and the remedial actions provided need to be documented. Taking this kind of action (as Jose's Vignette 2.1 illustrates) helps the learner to recognise the seriousness of their conduct. It also provides documentary evidence that the unsatisfactory performance has been recognised, and if appropriate, remedial action has been provided. Hopefully the individual will benefit from guidance and supervision, their practice will improve, and patient safety will be assured. Most learners are grateful that their mentor has cared sufficiently to help them. However, if they fail to respond to the documented action plan or carry on with the behaviour deemed unacceptable, then further action can be taken on the basis of the written evidence provided. The documentation provides the university with evidence of what support the learner has received.

Many practitioners express frustration at seeing learners that they have experienced as unsatisfactory remaining on their programme. As a result, they question the judgement of the university staff. However, without comprehensive and documented factual statements of a learner's behaviour, it is impossible for the university to deal with unsatisfactory behaviour effectively without being accused of discrimination or vindictiveness.

Educational responsibility

Supervising and supporting health care learners is an important part of the role of the registered practitioner. This is illustrated by the example of the Nursing and Midwifery Council 'Standards of Conduct, Performance and Ethics for Nurses and Midwives' (the Code 2008). This stipulates that a registered nurse or midwife 'must facilitate learners and others to develop their competence'. This places an important responsibility upon nurses and midwives who become mentors to share their professional knowledge and to promote their learner's professional development. The Code does not require them to engage in formal (classroom type) teaching or tutoring but to pass on their expertise. This knowledge is sometimes called 'finger-tip' knowledge or 'professional craft knowledge'. It is quite different from 'book knowledge' and is normally acquired after considerable practical experience. It is the kind of knowledge learners are thirsty to learn.

The American nurse researcher, Patricia Benner (Benner 1982), and colleagues (Benner et al. 1996) investigated how qualified nurses use their knowledge and found that 'expert' nurses had, over time, been able to internalise their reflections on earlier experiences and to develop a repertoire of strategies that worked in their specific field of practice. Building on earlier work with airline pilots by Dreyfus and Dreyfus (1986), Benner found that learning professional craft knowledge by newly registered nurses seemed to be on a continuum. Newly qualified nurses were identified as working like a novice who approached new experiences tentatively and needed to think deeply about every action as if it was a new experience. With accumulated experience and over time, they might progress through different stages of competence to become an expert. By contrast, experts were described as demonstrating an intuitive understanding of how to respond effectively and seemingly effortlessly to every clinical challenge. Expert practitioners seemed to have a repertoire of professional strategies, some of which were immediately transferable to other clinical settings, while other strategies needed to be re-shaped to meet the care needs of patients when encountered in a new setting. Benner's research indicates the complexity of developing professional expertise and the importance of its effective communication to novice practitioners particularly. Her research also illustrates how challenging it must be for learners to understand what they need to learn and how much they rely upon skilled practitioners to teach them both the elementary aspects of technical skill acquisition as well as the sophisticated nuances of professional practice that delivers effective and therapeutic care.

As a mentor and a registered practitioner, it is likely that you are also developing expertise in your own specific field of practice, and as research indicates, many mentors believe they can benefit from using teaching opportunities for their own professional development (Wisdom 2012). Throughout their placement career, learners will be exposed to practitioners at different stages in their development as experts.

One of the pioneers of nursing research, Carper (1975), classified expert nursing practice under four specific domains that she described as 'fundamental patterns of knowing'.

Carper's patterns of nursing knowledge

Carper's model of nursing provides a framework for understanding the complexity of nursing practice. She identified four patterns of nursing knowledge: the *empirical*, concerned with scientific knowledge associated with evidence-based practice, *aesthetic* knowledge, *personal* knowledge and *moral* knowledge. Empirical knowledge may be equated with formal research-based knowledge, commonly associated with medical practice, although more recently, much nursing research has been undertaken to provide a wealth of evidence to inform practice. From the literature, it appears that in the past, nurses rarely made use of research-based information that was available (Hamilton Smith 1972; Jones 1974; Wright 1975). With professional education now being at degree level, research understanding is a fundamental part of the curriculum.

Although focused on nursing practice, Carper's other three other forms of knowledge have relevance to all practitioners and perhaps require more detailed exploration and discussion, as they provide some insights to the kinds of knowledge that health and social care learners need to acquire.

Aesthetic knowledge

Carper's second pattern of knowledge was concerned with the *aesthetic* or art of nursing. She argued that the art of nursing can be expressed by creativity and style with which nurses plan and provide care that is both effective and satisfying. In skilful delivery of such care, the nurse would be acting in partnership with the patient in a holistic and problem-solving manner. Her actions are generated by applying a range of solutions to fit the particular needs of clients in a manner described by Argyris (1982) as Model II theories in use. Schön (1987) uses a similar notion of artistry to describe 'reflection in action', whereby practitioners build solutions to specific problems, which Schön calls knowledge in action rather than trying to fit a problem to ready-made solutions. Practising as a reflective practitioner requires different types of knowledge: the knowledge that there is the existence of a problem (or that the situation is different from normal), of how to assess the care needed, to plan its delivery, to deliver care skilfully (the outcome) and the breadth of knowledge and thinking, awareness and empathy that is being employed (process) and to evaluate its effectiveness.

These types of knowledge and behaviour appear similar to Heron's Experiential Knowledge (Heron 1981: 27), which he describes as difficult to codify or document. Transmission of such knowledge can only be gained through observation and experience (Eraut 1985: 120). This kind of experience is enhanced when accompanied by supervision with coaching through 'criticism' and comment that encourages the learner to approximate their performance towards an ideal standard. However, this kind of coaching can only be effective when the learner and coach feel confident and when there is a bond of trust in the relationship. What these researchers are describing is the importance to learners of being able to work alongside an accomplished practitioner and being able to 'pick up' the techniques including the use of language, body posture and self as well as the knowledge that is inherently informing the activity. Vignette 2.3 provides an example of how this can work.

Vignette 2.3   Working and learning together: mentor and learner

Cherie is working with her co-mentor, Max, in her second community placement. Today, they are running a weekly clinic for new mothers bringing their babies for a regular checkup. Cherie has little experience of handling toddlers or babies and is quite nervous about this experience. From the beginning of the clinic, Max took the lead, talking to the mothers and measuring and placing their babies on the weighing scales. After an hour, he handed a sleeping baby to Cherie and asked her to take the measurements. Cherie was a bit surprised but without thinking took the baby, placed it comfortably on the scales and proceeded to carry out the task without the baby stirring. Over the next hour, Cherie took charge of the baby weighing and measurements, while Max talked to the mothers and checked that Cherie was managing safely. By coffee time, Cherie was feeling much more confident and was pleased that Max suggested that they took turns to weigh the babies and talk to the mothers.

Points to ponder:

What skills do you think Max was demonstrating to Cherie?
What do you think Cherie might have learned from this experience?
Do you think this way of working impeded the normal pace of the clinic significantly, if at all?

It looks as though Cherie and Max have developed a trusting relationship, and Max was aware of Cherie's nervousness about handling small babies. By role modelling how to do it and then giving Cherie the opportunity to undertake this important part of the morning's work, this increased her confidence to the extent that she was able to make a genuine contribution. As a result, her confidence and her professional skills were increased. This kind of supportive supervision in a democratic relationship is vital to helping learners achieve professional maturity in an environment where she was able to make mistakes without dire consequences to either herself or their clients (Marsick 1987). It is likely that Max and Cherie discussed some of the issues that arose from their work together that morning, such as whether the babies were developing normally, how each mother was coping and whether there were any signs of difficulties within the family, from other siblings or from social factors such as housing or nutrition. Having a discussion such as this broadens Cherie's understanding of the value of the clinic as well as helping her to develop both her observational and intellectual skills, making the morning's work less routine and more of a valuable learning experience, as well as providing insights into the value of Max's work.

Personal knowledge

Carper's third pattern of knowing is *personal knowledge*. She relates this to Buber's perspective of I–Thou relationships (Buber 1937) where the 'other' is encountered as an extension of self, rather than as being an object. In a sense, this is what we were discussing earlier in this chapter. The philosophy is related to principles of Quantum physics and to what Quantum psychologists describe as the inter-connectedness of all earth's organisms, the influence of each action being reverberated throughout the physical and spiritual environment (Zohar 1990). Traditional cultures have retained this sense of interconnectedness with the universe, as have people who subscribe to the Buddhist faith. This is reflected in the Judaic, Christian and Muslim faiths where people are experienced as brothers or sisters. Professional standards from regulatory organisations are designed to establish practices where each member of the community, including patients/clients as well as the staff, recognise their inter-dependence and thus their interconnectedness. Thus, the practitioner opens themself up to recognising the individual (patient or learner) as an extension of self with shared feelings and life experiences. In such environments, the educational or care relationship becomes therapeutic and effective. To achieve this kind of personal knowledge, as defined by Carper, further exploration of self by the practitioner (whether a learner or a registered practitioner) is necessary and can only effectively take place in a supportive and caring environment.

Points to ponder:

- How might this philosophy of I–Thou be reflected in your own practice, as a clinician and as a mentor?
- To what extent do policies concerned with equal rights and non-discriminatory practice reflect this philosophy of interconnectedness?

The Moral Component

Carper's fourth pattern of knowing is 'the moral component of knowing, or ethics'. She describes this as the morality of nursing, which goes beyond simply knowing the ethical codes of the discipline. It includes all voluntary actions that are deliberate and subject to the judgement of right and wrong. Berthold (1968) argues that making such choices of this nature is subject to personal values. Personal choices may in turn be affected by empirical evidence, or by ethical or moral beliefs and cultural perspectives. Practitioners working in our globalised and thus multi-cultural society will inevitably face challenges to their assumptions about moral and ethical conduct. Such challenges can lead to dissonance/personal conflicts. Recognising this, the Nursing and Midwifery Council's 2008 Code sets standards for ethical conduct and behaviour.

Researching nursing in the 1960s, a psychologist (Menzies 1970) discovered that the traditional hierarchical structure of nursing that existed in the 1960s militated against decision-making and accountability. Her work was further substantiated in the 1980s by Fretwell (1982), who found that learners were unlikely to learn in clinical settings that were hierarchical and impersonal. By contrast, the professional model of nursing practice described by Carper gives autonomy and accountability to the nurse (Manthey 1980). Manthey argues that nurses who are able to respond reflexively to their patients and to learners are in a better position to observe and practise decision-making skills. The movement towards making the patient or client the centre of the decision-making process in partnership with the nurse gives dignity and autonomy to both the patient and the nurse. In the same way, you can involve your learner as a friend and be sensitive to their needs while being clear about your own professional responsibilities.

Professional accountability

By virtue of your professional Registration, you acknowledge your commitment to practise according to the ethical and moral standards enshrined by the Code described by your professional statutory organisation. Essentially, ethical and moral practice entails maintaining and developing your professional knowledge so that you can deliver the best quality of care to those patients for whom you are responsible and accountable. Practising as a 'virtuous practitioner' (Whaite 2003) entails the characteristics of courage, honesty and loyalty. It requires great courage to stand up to the bully or to the colleague whose practice is unethical and causes others to suffer, especially courageous when colleagues are too afraid to be supportive. Too many public investigations and reports into unsatisfactory standards of care illustrate how difficult confronting bad practice can be. By omitting to complain and raise the alarum, practitioners are equally guilty of the neglect and malpractice that they inadvertently condoned through their silence. Developing a habitual response to take the 'right' action in practice fosters an environment where high standards of care become the norm. For example, the Nursing and Midwifery Council has published a paper providing guidelines for nurses and midwives facing such situations: *Raising and Escalating Concerns: Guidance for Nurses and Midwives* (Nursing and Midwifery Council 2010a). Throughout your career as a registered nurse, you are accountable for the care delivered to patients under your care. This maxim applies, even if you are not the person who actually delivers the care but the one who is supervising and therefore supporting learners and staff who are the care deliverers. If you identify that a learner or a colleague is acting in an unprofessional manner, you have a professional responsibility to discuss their behaviour with the individual immediately and to notify your own line manager (and the person responsible for the learner) of your concerns. It is also important that you document the incident and a report of your discussion with the individual immediately. The purpose of this is twofold: essentially to enable the individual to change their behaviour and, if necessary, to receive further training. Second, you need to fulfil your professional obligations as a registered practitioner to protect the public and to meet the requirements of the Professional Code of Conduct, Performance and Ethics.

Defining negligence

Negligence is defined as 'omitting to do something that a reasonable person, guided by those considerations that ordinarily regulate the conduct of human affairs, would do, or (by contrast) to do something that a reasonable person would *not* do'. Negligent behaviour may be perpetrated by a colleague or by a learner who is under your supervision or by practitioners working on their own. In either situation, you are professionally accountable.

Proving negligent action is difficult and requires documented evidence. Essentially, it requires three aspects:

- evidence that the accused person (the defendant) is responsible for the care delivery to the injured party (i.e., has a duty of care towards the plaintiff);
- the injured party (the plaintiff) must prove that there has been a breach of that duty;
- that the injured party (the plaintiff) suffered consequential damage as a result of the defendant's behaviour.

By law, the responsibility for proving that negligence has taken place is the responsibility of the injured party (the plaintiff), which may be difficult if that person is frail or confused. As a result, the registered practitioner has a responsibility to act on their behalf. Keeping accurate and comprehensive records of care planning and its delivery is vital to ensure that a fair and full investigation can be conducted, even when it may take place several years after the event. The Nursing and Midwifery Council Code *Standards of Conduct, Performance and Ethics*, for example, requires registrants to keep and maintain accurate records. The NMC provides a publication, *Record Keeping: Guidance for Nurses and Midwives* (Nursing and Midwifery Council 2009), that can be downloaded from their web site (www.nmc-uk.org).

Most nursing and midwifery learners undertake the rigorous period of study and practice because they have a vocation to help others and to do good in society. As with every profession and every walk of life, there are people who contradict such aspirations and one unsatisfactory learner can cause staff to feel antipathy towards all learners.

If an act of negligence has been perpetrated by a learner under your supervision, you are accountable. To protect yourself, you need to provide evidence that the learner was capable of delivering the care without your direct supervision and was given the appropriate preparation and guidance for its delivery. This means that the care plan for the patient was clearly documented and reviewed appropriately, and that you had satisfied yourself that the learner was able to deliver all aspects of the delegated care safely and effectively. The subsequent chapters will explore some strategies for monitoring and evaluating learners' readiness to practise under distant supervision.

Learners' perspective on supportive relationships

Entering an unfamiliar setting and not knowing what they will meet is daunting for every thoughtful adult. Many learners have come into health or social care professions after successful careers in other settings and so carry a self image that can be easily shaken unless they are helped to feel welcomed and valued. Melia (1987) describing nursing learners pre-Project 2000 experiences in Scotland identified how much time learners spent trying to 'fit in' to the clinical team and to 'learn the rules' that would enable them to 'get by' and to get a good report. Despite changes to the curriculum and the institution of professional standards for learner support in their placements, the literature is rich with accounts of the difficulties that nursing learners encounter (Nolan 1998; Levett-Jones and Lathlean 2008; Henderson et al. 2011) and how such difficulties affect their learning. Despite preparing for their career by undertaking work-experience in a clinical setting such as a care home or with people who have disabilities, learners still need to be welcomed and to be given time to adjust to each new placement. As the literature cited above demonstrates the quality of their sponsor and mentor is the most important factor in determining whether learners learn during their placement and whether they remain in their chosen profession, as the following indicate:

> It wasn't what I'd expected. It was a big culture shock really. I think I expected people to support people more, a bit more friendly. . . . . If this is what nursing is, I thought I didn't really want to do it. . . . . I suppose I expected people to be more caring and understanding and support each other' Jack (in Spouse 2003b: 77)

As a result of his experiences with these clinical staff Jack made poor progress and received unsatisfactory reports. In the end he decided to leave his general nursing programme and was advised to go into mental health nursing from which he successfully graduated. Sadly, his experiences were not unique as the following learners describe:

> Oh at first I felt as though I wasn't wanted there because my mentor was ill and everyone was going' Well, who's going to have the learner?' Well I can't have her because I've got this and this to do.' And I felt like going home in the end and in the end the only reason I didn't was because I'd got up at 6 am to get there. But when my mentor was there it was really good and she knew what I wanted to know. Marie (in Spouse 2003b: 53)

Ruth has a similar observation about what it felt like to be a learner:

> I almost feel that I'm nudging my way in with my elbows out. You've got the staff in a circle and the learners are on the outside and you're trying to push in between and say 'Here I am, if

you want me I'm here'. I find it very disheartening at times. (In another placement I felt accepted) and valued; to a minor point that I've got my name up on the board . . . Ruth (in Spouse 2003b: 112/113)

These three learners are describing situations that seem to be part of every learners' experience of going into unfamiliar clinical settings. As Marie and Ruth explain, when they had a mentor who took the time to get to know them and to assess their learning needs it reduced their anxiety and increased their confidence. Ruth's experience of having her name on the Work board where the patients' nurses were identified, was a public statement of her contribution to the overall workload and thus she was identified as a legitimate member of the clinical team with a role to play.

The process of feeling accepted into the clinical team includes being allowed to reciprocate the efforts of their mentor by undertaking minor tasks that contribute to the workload:

But when you're actually getting your hands into the 'muck' so as to speak, and getting doing things you feel as though you're more use. Because otherwise if you are not doing anything you feel as if you're wasting your time and their, the ward's time. . . . You know what's the point of being there? Marie (in Spouse 2003b, 53)

Engaging learners in activities that contribute to the overall workload and provide them with much needed and appropriate experience allows everyone to benefit.

Models of mentoring/supervision

Working in partnership with one or more learners at different levels of their programme can be a demanding and exhausting process. The number of learners coming through each clinical setting can seem endless. The rewards can be high when supporting a learner who develops confidence and is able to make a strong contribution to the overall work of the team. By contrast, some learners struggle to find their feet and require a great deal of encouragement and time, draining the mentor of energy. So, how can you as a mentor find ways to both support the learner and protect yourself from burnout while ensuring learners receive consistent supervision and effective feedback?

Within the relationship, there are several strategies and processes that can be of help. There are also structures that can be developed within the clinical setting to support different approaches to mentoring, some of which build upon existing care-delivery structures such as team nursing or team midwifery, primary nursing or key-worker: the one-to-one relationship; the team mentoring process; the mentor and co-mentor; peer mentoring support. Choosing which structure to use depends upon the way in which learners come to the placement. If they come in blocks of time and are on the same duty roster as their mentor, a one-to-one relationship will offer the best opportunities for close working. However, if learners come at irregular intervals and can negotiate their shifts, then a team mentoring approach or having a co-mentor might ensure they receive consistent supervision. It also makes effective communication between supervisors more likely.

One-to-one mentoring

Learners allocated to their personal or key mentor need that person to be available to them when they are on duty. Their mentor needs to plan and discuss their work plan for the shift with the learner as well as having time to debrief the learner at the end of the shift. Documentation of the learner's progress and response to any action plans is best undertaken by this key mentor. As a result, a relationship based on trust and mutual respect can develop, whereby giving a receiving feedback can be a natural part of the process.

Co-mentoring

Co-mentoring is a valuable strategy of ensuring a learner is supported in the absence of their key mentor or if that person has a role that makes one-to-one working difficult. It is also a helpful way of introducing a new practitioner to the mentoring role so they receive help and guidance. It can also be helpful if a learner has had difficulty in the past and is likely to need quite focused support during the placement. Having two people who are collaborating to support the learner gives the learner the best opportunity to make progress as well as to have appropriate feedback, providing communication between all three people is good!

Setting up a co-mentoring partnership means that the three people need to have a preliminary meeting together where they can agree on:

- the learner's learning needs and priorities;
- the plan of actions;
- the rotation of collaborative working;
- dates for interim feedback and documentation of progress.

The advantages of two registered practitioners working together to support a learner are that the burden is spread, and the risk of emotional exhaustion is reduced. Co-mentoring increases the support available to the learner. The disadvantage of co-mentoring is the inevitable risk of the learner not receiving effective support from either mentor owing to a failure in communication.

Team mentoring

Team mentoring relies upon the structures used to manage care. If the registered practitioners work in teams, a learner can be allocated to the team. This enables the learner to work any shift under the direct supervision of the team member on duty. Each team member recognises the learner as being part of their team and their duty of care towards the learner. Arrangements for learner supervision may be with the team leader who takes overall responsibility, or for delegating specific responsibility to a named team member. Ensuring the learner is capable of carrying out patient care and providing learning opportunities that extend and challenge their knowledge makes for effective practice, beneficial not only to the team but also to the patients. Team mentorship can also provide support for the mentor, as it provides a forum for discussion and for anxieties to be explored and resolved. There is, however, a risk that the newcomer 'slips through the net', and no one helps them or monitors their performance, believing someone else is giving the support. Learners need to know who is responsible for documenting their progress and writing reports.

The process of assessing, planning and documenting the learner's needs and progress must also be undertaken by the responsible key mentor within the team. It may be that learners are given a learning plan (rather like a patient care plan) so that the team can contribute to the documentation and agree on the progress reports.

As with co-mentoring, the advantage of team mentoring is that learners receive support from a team member whenever they are on duty. It also gives the key mentor support in the supervision and decision-making processes. The system can fail if there are poor communication structures and processes between team members, and as a result both learners and staff can suffer. With effective policies in operation, everyone knows what is happening, and good communication can ensure the learner and the staff members benefit without feeling under pressure.

Peer mentorship

Buddying or peer mentorship that has been planned ensures the newcomer has a contact within the community of practice. An imaginative New Zealand project developed by the academic team prepared and supervised third-year learners buddying first years during their first placement. They found it could be advantageous to a senior learner to mentor a junior learner (McDougall & Beattie 1997; Yates et al. 1997). Their evaluations indicated that both groups of learners benefited from the experience. Third years were able to consolidate their knowledge, as well as develop supervision skills, and first years reported feeling able to provide care that was safe (Isles & Freer 1999). However, buddying systems should not be undertaken instead of permanent placement members, as there is always a risk that either the third year or the junior learner is too weak without realising it and needs more experienced help. Another risk is that the structure can create insiders (permanent staff) and outsiders (learners).

On the positive side, buddying a less experienced colleague can enable the more experienced learner to externalise their knowledge and to recognise areas of deficit through the process of explaining, procedures, specialist practice or theories (Wood 1998). Many people prefer to ask questions of a peer because they are afraid of appearing rude if they ask of a senior colleague (Spouse 2003b), and so peer mentorship makes it easier for learners to challenge each other's knowledge and learn how to ask questions.

All of these four models of supervision provide structures that engage newcomers in the community of practice and in its daily activities, particularly if the management style is democratic and fully engages all learners (Fretwell 1985; Edmond 2001).

Approaches to mentoring

In the 1980s, the American nurse researcher, Darling (1985), investigated the approaches to mentoring newly registered nurses and classified her findings into six key approaches. Some of the approaches were helpful and developmental; others were counter-productive and destructive to the well-being of the neophyte nurse.

In the United Kingdom, Gray and Smith conducted a longitudinal study with 17 pre-registration nursing learners to find out what they believed were the qualities of an effective mentor during the first year of their programme (Gray & Smith 2000). They identified four specific characteristics:

- *supporter* – gives advice, sorts out problems or worries, can be relied upon as an ally and a friend, has a genuine interest in the learner and is respected by peers;
- *guide and teacher* – the essential role – takes time to explain things, to organise and arrange visits; has realistic expectations of the learner; is a role model; facilitates the learner to observe different aspects of the patient care pathway, to practise under direct supervision and to have opportunities to practise with distant supervision; gives prompt and regular feedback on their performance; is a good communicator;
- *supervisor* – allows gradual development of independence;
- *assessor* – takes time to be involved in assessing their learning needs and their progress.

These findings support an Australian study (Hart and Rotem 1994) investigating senior undergraduate nursing learners' perceptions of learning opportunities in the clinical setting. Feeling accepted by the clinical staff, working with a practitioner who was familiar with the clinical setting and having opportunities to question practice were significant influences on learners' learning.

Several earlier, North American studies (Mogan and Knox 1987; Windsor 1987) investigated the characteristics of effective clinical instructors and came to the same conclusions. All these studies identified mentors who failed to support learners tended to lack the necessary clinical and educational skills and were often unhappy in their role. Darling (1985) labelled such mentors as toxic. Their attitudes reflected a range of behaviours from avoidance and dumping to blocking and destroying their learner. Darling described the dumpers as mentors who dump their learner in at the deep end with little or no help. Sometimes this is due to a lack of understanding of what the terms 'adult learning' and 'supernumerary' means for the learner.

Avoiders tend to leave the learner to sink or swim, while the 'blockers' refuse to meet their needs by failing to keep them informed or providing appropriate experience. The destroyers tended to undermine their learner confidence either by overt criticism or by a lack of feedback. It is possible that when you were a learner, you encountered mentors like these or have noticed some of these characteristics in colleagues. If you have a colleague who behaves like this, it is possible that they need help.

Emotional labour and mentoring

Research by several writers investigating mentor experiences in the United Kingdom (for example, Atkins and Williams 1995; Wisdom 2012) indicates that being a mentor is satisfying and professionally rewarding. They also suggest that mentors become exhausted by the constant stream of learners. So, how might you be able to look after yourself while enjoying the benefits?

Working in health care imposes a high demand on emotional health despite the strong commitment from most practitioners. Mackay's research found that despite the stress, most nurses derived enormous job satisfaction from supporting people through difficult times in their life (Mackay 1989). Engaging in a vocation such as health care with so much commitment and respect for others echoes the work of writers such as Martin Buber (1937), an Hasidic philosopher who believed that human existence depended upon individual relationships. The highest form of relationship depended upon recognition of the 'other' without prejudice and as an equal. He describes this relationship as the I–Thou relationship and as being the most fulfilling and appropriate when working in partnership with others. Carl Rogers, the American psychotherapist and influential educationalist, advocated a similar approach in his person-centred therapy, which he also applied to education (Rogers 1961; 1983). Buber and Rogers argue that personal development and thus learning can best be achieved through openness to the other and a willingness to acknowledge their world. Campbell (1984), writing about the ministry of religion in particular, describes 'skilled companionship' as the process of being sensitive to another person's needs and to being willing to engage in them. The notable American nurse and philosopher, Jean Watson (2009), uses similar arguments in her model of 'patient-centred care'.

Successful skilled companionship entails a level of objectivity and understanding of the professional boundaries that enable the relationship to be genuinely and mutually developmental. Such relationships can inevitably create tensions for the facilitator (or mentor) that Carl Rogers recognises. He argues that by being aware of personal tensions and taking notice of their cause and effect, the facilitator can be genuinely developmental by offering insights to the other of the effects of their behaviour (Rogers 1961). From Rogers' perspective, being genuinely sensitive to the 'other' requires insight and openness, and is a skill that takes time to develop. Opportunities to reflect back to the 'other' may not always be available or appropriate, which can leave both parties feeling upset: for the 'other,' because they are likely to recognise the incongruence between actions and feelings of their facilitator, and for the facilitator, who may be feeling disgruntled.

Another researcher, who investigated how airline hostesses and debt collectors manage to maintain a comportment that is both friendly and 'professional' irrespective of the behaviour of their clients, described the behaviour as 'emotional labour' (Hochshild 1983). Like Carl Rogers, Arlee Russell Hochshild discovered that to achieve emotional congruence, 'actors' need to balance genuine feelings of concern with actions. When they pretend to themselves or to their 'client' they have feelings that are dissonant with their genuine feeling, 'burnout' can ensue. Working in situations where sensitivity to emotions is important, requires intelligence and training of the practitioners so that they do not suffer from emotional burnout. Hochshild categorised the responses to emotional labour into what she called 'feeling rules' (see Box 2.1).

Box 2.1   Emotional labour and feeling rules.

1. Make actions congruent with personal feelings
2. Feelings and actions may not be congruent because of the nature of the situation
3. The recipient of the interaction should believe there is congruence between the actions and the underlying feelings
4. Achieving congruence can be challenging
5. Role strain and self destruction will ensue if there is a conflict between actions and feelings
6. The consequence of 5 is emotional burnout unless effective coping strategies are developed

Rogers and Hochschild both argue for practitioners to develop the ability to recognise their feelings through reflection on incidents that cause dissonance and on the effect that it is having on their own personal being. This can be helped by asking such questions as:

- 'Is it the behaviour of the person that is creating my sense of unease or is it to do with the personality of the individual?'
- 'Why am I feeling this about the person?'
- 'What is it about them that is so familiar that I feel uncomfortable?'
- 'Are my feelings due to my own pre-conscious anxieties (anger or whatever), or is it genuinely to do with this person's behaviour?'

Having arrived at some preliminary solution to such questions, the facilitator is in a stronger position to make a response that is congruent with their feelings while being facilitative to the genuine needs of the other.

From her research into how British nursing learners develop the ability to cope with emotionally challenging situations, Smith (1992) and Smith and Gray (2001) found that learners watched how other nurses in the practice setting dealt with difficult situations. They would adapt their approach if it matched their own philosophy. The following learners' accounts from research by Spouse (2003a, b) indicate how they achieved this:

> She was really good when a chap came in who was dying, and he was being a pain . . . quite arrogant and offensive. Maybe it was his insecurities coming out, but she was really good with the relatives and spent a lot of time with them afterwards. Jack (in Spouse 2003a, b, 84)

> The nurses on there who I thought were really good were the ones who treated the children with respect and didn't patronise them. They let them know what was going on and tried to reflect back to them why their behaviour pattern wasn't appropriate. . . . . The nurses I admired were the ones who were able to do that and able to deal with the crisis situation swiftly and without any undue alarm to anyone else. Nicola (in Spouse 2003a, b, 69)

Giving learners the opportunity to discuss their observations and experiences toward the end of each shift provides you with opportunities to correct any false impressions as well as giving both of you the means to debrief from events that might have been upsetting. Sharing experiences in this way increases mutual understanding and trust. It is also important that you and your own colleagues are facilitated to share your concerns and worries in a supportive environment. Some clinical settings have weekly group debriefing sessions facilitated by a mental-health practitioner. Sessions like this can help colleagues to appreciate each other's emotional needs and improve the mental health of everyone in the team, as well as creating a collegiate atmosphere.

Summary

In this chapter, we have explored some of the principles for successfully supporting learners in your own professional setting. We have proposed that entering a seemingly tightly knit community of practitioners can be very daunting for a learner, and the quality of the relationship they can establish with their supervisor influences their success or failure, not only for the duration of their placement but also potentially for their career.

As a practitioner and supervisor of learners, you have a professional responsibility towards your clients to protect them from harm by action or by omission to act. Your duty of care thus requires you to ensure that your learner is safe to practise under distant supervision, but only after you have established their level of competency and have allocated appropriate experiences for them to further develop their professional knowledge. You can achieve this by creating and regularly reviewing your agreed learning plan with your supervisee. Through your personalised support, most learners will flourish. However, there are a few learners who, for whatever reason, have difficulties and they often benefit from an even more structured approach. For these learners, it is vitally important to document their progress or lack of progress in detail and their response to the help they are given. By taking this kind of care with a weak learner, you will be saving yourself considerable time and worry, both for the present and for future colleagues and their patients.

The different models of supervision and the approach that you may take also have a strong impact on your learner. Your own personal well-being is important, and so having access to emotional and professional support is essential to ensuring that the supervision process is mutually beneficial.

Chapter 3

The workplace as a learning environment: structures and sources of support and supervision

Jenny Spouse

Introduction

This chapter will explore what is traditionally known as the 'Learning Environment'. We will explore the idea from the macro (the social and physical environment) and the micro (the inter-personal and educational relationships). The macro learning environment is concerned with policies and protocols, both official and unofficial, that influence the workplace setting and in particular how learning and learners are treated within the clinical environment. The quality of the setting as a learning environment is also influenced by the physical geography in which the working experience is offered as well as important structures such as support systems, availability of human and, importantly, material resources.

The second essential component of successful learning in the workplace is the quality of the micro-environment. The leadership and philosophy of the team influence the personal interactions, relationships and working practices that make up the micro-environment. This chapter will explore in some depth these two aspects of the learning environment, how they affect learning and what you can do to enhance and promote effective learning for the novice and the newcomer.

We shall explore these two aspects of the workplace using vignettes that illustrate the different dimensions of a learning environment. The chapter includes the following:

- the concept of the learning environment, micro and macro factors, the influence of geography;
- policies and protocols and the learning environment. their effect on structures such as client group, staffing levels and skill mix; number and range of visiting learners, delivery of care, reception and management of newcomers, professional education, interactions with health and social care team members.
- supporting visiting learners;

Practice-Based Learning in Nursing, Health and Social Care: Mentorship, Facilitation and Supervision,
First Edition. Ian Scott and Jenny Spouse.
© 2013 John Wiley & Sons, Ltd. Published 2013 by John Wiley & Sons, Ltd.

- protocols – using evidence; protocols in delivery of client care and how their use influences the quality of learning; the human contribution to learning; influences of other professionals within the clinical environment;
- collaborative learning among the professions;
- audit tool for placement learning environment.

Concept of a learning environment, micro and macro factors

What is a learning environment?

The introduction to this chapter implies that a workplace can be experienced as a good or a poor place to learn by its staff, and by anyone else who contributes to the function of the setting, including visiting practitioners and learners. An effective learning environment is created from several structures and processes (see Table 3.1). From Table 3.1, you will see that structures include the physical organisation of the setting, its geography and availability of non-human resources as well as suitable storage facilities. Professional structures influence not only the ability of the team to function but also the ability of visiting learners to benefit from their placement. These professional structures include policies and protocols (the human and social structures), such as the workforce, its size, the skill mix, and the number and range of regular visitors who have professional responsibilities towards the client group as well as the visiting learners from different professions. Policies, whether formal or informal, also influence the social relationships between staff, their opportunities to meet formally and informally; the volume of learners who enter the setting, the duration of their stay and their level of knowledge on entry; the purpose of the setting, client numbers, levels of dependency, turnover and time available to attend to each client; and opportunities for staff to obtain continuing education, and for learners to extend their professional knowledge. Table 3.1 illustrates many of these structures, and you might like to consider how the different aspects influence the quality of learning. A copy is available in Appendix 3.1 in the form of an audit questionnaire that you can use to evaluate your own workplace.

Influence of geography on the learning environment

The easiest kind of work-setting to describe is a geographical area managed by one person, staffed by a core team of workers, with visiting practitioners and peripatetic learners. You can imagine this definition applying to a shop or a factory, a hospital ward or department, a community health centre, social-work practice or dental practice and so on. In these settings, the geographical area is clearly demarcated, and members of the team are always 'visible' and accessible during the shift. Leadership of the team is usually stable, and the geography provides opportunities for frequent social interactions that strengthen the bond and understanding between team members. Considering the geography of a different kind of learning environment, such as that created by a team of people working from an agency in the community, illustrates how more difficult communication and regular interactions are likely to be.

Table 3.1   Dimensions of the learning environment.

Physical aspects	Social aspects	Professional aspects	Philosophical and educational aspects
Geography – is it a compact and discrete environment, or is it spread over a wide geographical area?	Staffing: is it adequate and of the correct skill mix for the work of the setting, including the number of peripatetic learners, for example, do professional staff undertake clerical work in the absence of a clerk or vice versa? Does the skill mix account for the increased workload of learner supervision?	Are the purpose and the function of the workplace clear and respected, that is, are staffing and skill mix appropriate for the nature of clients? Are staff adequately and appropriately prepared for the nature of work and for the clients? Are staff appropriately prepared to support learners?	Is there a mission statement, or statement of beliefs, agreed and documented that informs the work of the team? Is there evidence that this influences all aspects of practice? Is work allocated on the basis of capability and as a means of supervised professional development?
Is the area adequate for the function of the team? Are the facilities appropriate for the client group at all stages of their care?	Are there structures in place to ensure staff meet regularly and frequently for peer support, and for exchange of information, for problem-solving?	Is the breadth of professional support appropriate for the client group, that is, are the appropriate clinical specialists available to provide advice and support to the clients and the staff?	Are clients' wishes identified and respected? Are clients treated according to the highest of professional standards? Are clients and their carers invited to evaluate their care?
Are there adequate storage facilities for the resources and is access to them appropriate?	Is the quality of communication effective between internal staff and senior management of the institution and with visiting staff?	Are protocols and professional practices implemented to the highest standards, and are these audited on a regular and frequent basis?	Is staff education an important and continuous part of the overall function of the team? Are staff encouraged to implement new practices and thinking?
Is communication between staff facilitated by the physical resources, for example, internet access, handheld systems?	Is there effective leadership within the clinical team? Are the relationships between the different professional groups associated with the work focus effective and constructive?	Are continuing education and use of evidence-based practices promoted and implemented? Are the equipment and other resources appropriate for the nature of work? Is there an agreement about the number, range and skill mix of visiting learners?	Does the range of visiting learners reflect the available skill mix to ensure their adequate support and supervision? Are there regular planned opportunities for learners from different professions to learn and work together?

Table 3.1 *(cont'd)*

Physical aspects	Social aspects	Professional aspects	Philosophical and educational aspects
Are there places where staff can meet each other both formally and informally?	Is there effective management of the team? Are there effective structures to ensure policies and protocols are implemented?	Are visiting learners encouraged to participate fully in the work of the team based on their assessed capability? Are learners encouraged to participate in case conferences and team meetings?	Are there effective policies on the support and supervision of visiting learners? Is staff workload adjusted when supervising a learner? Is learner feedback encouraged and acted upon?
Can equipment or other resources be ordered and delivered effectively and on time?	Do staff have clear and effective guidelines and avenues of management when dealing with difficult and challenging situations?	Are support services effective? Are there regular visits from other members of the health and social care team to support the client-care package?	Are there written guidelines and documented learning opportunities for visiting learners made available to them prior to arrival?

So, a team working in the community from 'agency' offices may not work in a physical environment that is tightly demarcated in the same manner as a hospital ward, and it will be the learning environment created by individual practitioners that will have a greater impact on visiting learners. Despite this, the practitioners will still be affected by the same kinds of local structures: policies and processes, inter-relationships, workload, access to resources. These in turn will influence the quality of relationship and effectiveness practitioners enjoy with their 'consumer group'. Wherever a learner is sent for professional experience, they are entering a learning environment of some kind.

Point to ponder – the effect of geography:
Having read these descriptions of a geographical learning environment, consider your own workplace and jot down your answers to the following questions:

• How would you describe the geography of your work setting?
• To what extent are the boundaries physically defined?
• What are the core influences on the way in which you work and learn?
• What do you find to be the most and least frustrating aspects of your workplace and why?
• What are the core aspects that hinder or promote your own professional development and learning?

The geography of a workplace influences opportunities for informal peer support and thus team building. Managers with practitioners who work away from their administrative centre in widespread community settings have to work harder to develop a supportive team spirit that fosters sharing of good practice or discussing practice dilemmas. While those working in a discrete area such as a hospital department or a general practice are less likely to have this challenge, small, stable and tightly knit communities tend to have stronger personal relationships and better opportunities for discussing issues. They are also at risk of developing rigid and entrenched attitudes, including factions, that are difficult to resolve or that can deter newcomers from entering. Visiting learners entering either work setting will progress only if they are welcomed and given sponsorship or if they are befriended by a senior member of the team. Newcomers need this kind of hosting – introduced to the other members of the community and the informal rules as well as being shown how to find their way around and where to find the 'tools of the trade'. Some authors have described a discrete group of practitioners sharing similar professional interests as a 'Community of Practice' (Lave & Wenger 1991; Wenger 1998).

Geography also has an influence on access to resources such as equipment, information and peer support. Working as a small team in a large geographical area requires careful organisational structures to ensure that the equipment necessary is always on hand where needed. For example, a client requiring lifting and bathing aids needs to be assessed before the equipment is delivered and installed into their home. The chain of people organising and supplying such equipment need to have an effective support system that ensures the processes take place efficiently and rapidly, so that the client receives the most effective care that they need. The alternative is wasted time and energy as well as frustration for the practitioner and greater immobility or even unnecessary death for the client.

Working in a hospital ward or department, such equipment is normally available as an essential standard. By contrast, often minor but important articles may be difficult to obtain because of a poor system of stock taking and commissioning. Similarly, without policies and structures that ensure there is an effective maintenance system, including sufficient skilled staff, the equipment is more likely to fail. The result will be time lost hunting down the necessary equipment or trying to get the equipment repaired, or incorrect procedures being used, with the risk of danger to clients and staff, and inappropriate practice being learned.

Peer understanding and co-operation are achieved by staff working closely together. The same applies to visiting learners working in a one-to-one relationship with a professional colleague. Learners will receive a higher quality of support than those who are left to work on their own or with a colleague whose skills and knowledge are limited.

From reading the above paragraphs, you can see that the learning environment is influenced by a range of issues associated with the physical structure of the workplace. Many of these issues can be managed by effective policies and protocols that may be formal, developed by a governing body of representatives guided by examples of best practice, or informal, developed from custom and practice or by an individual or small group of individuals and which may not reflect research-based evidence.

Points to ponder – search and find:

- Where are your organisational policies and protocols kept in your workplace setting?
- Who designed them and when?
- How do these policies and protocols affect your working?
- How are visiting learners and new staff introduced to them?
- How often are the policies and protocols reviewed?
- Who reviews your protocols?

Policies and protocols and the learning environment

Staffing and skill mix

Creating policies to determine staffing levels and skill mix are difficult to get right in health and social care settings because of the incredible variables in workload, volume of patients/clients and their degree of dependence. Government policies regarding education of health care practitioners, the number of learners, the availability of post-qualification education and training, and the funding of health and social care delivery systems all inevitably influence the skill mix. Internal policies, influenced by external funding, affect decisions about the ratio of professionally prepared staff to assistant practitioners or other minimally prepared staff. Another factor in determining staffing levels is the availability and retention of qualified staff, who are often more mobile and perhaps only stay for a relatively short time, while assistant practitioners tend to be local, cheaper to employ and less mobile, making them a more attractive source of labour. Working as a mentor in an environment with low professional, peer support is challenging, especially when coupled with an increasingly expanded role and a diverse range of patients/clients to manage. Unlike medical and social-work programmes for example, staffing policies in health care settings rarely include allowances for supporting nursing and midwifery learners. As a result, most staff providing supervision are expected to increase their workload in order to accommodate visiting learners, with the inevitable consequences of role strain and ill health, leading to sickness or absence from work, as well as disillusioned learners. Many qualified staff leave their profession despite their love of the job, because they cannot cope with its stresses and lack of peer support.

Developing a policy on staffing levels and skill mix is one of the hardest aspects to get right, and yet it influences so many aspects of the quality of outcome and client satisfaction as well as the long-term viability of the workforce. For a staffing policy to be effective, there needs to be access to a range of resources, including adequate funding and availability of a range of skilled practitioners, a stable workforce and a consistent client population. Another aspect of staffing policies that is vital to quality is a belief in ongoing staff development beyond the routine statutory requirements. Creating an environment where staff are encouraged to investigate, review and refresh their practice is an essential step towards high standards of practice as well as a means to demonstrate appreciation of each one of them as individuals. Many health and social care organisations do not enjoy such necessities, as they are often struggling to meet minimum standards. Nevertheless, it is important to have a comprehensive policy on staffing, as it can be used to bid for increased resources, or as an argument for failure to meet targets.

Developing policies

Policies that influence the management of the workplace are normally developed by teams of people, either within the setting or, if it is a large organisation, by a committee made up of representatives from all the staff. Such policies are used to design local structures such as levels of staffing, skill mix, working hours, dining facilities and so on. They are often influenced by an underlying philosophy or belief system, which may be of a mechanistic or industrial type model that can be quantitatively measured, such as rate of turnover, bed occupancy, waiting times and hospital length of stay. Alternatively, decisions may be driven by quality standards that are more difficult to quantify and are evaluated qualitatively, such as client satisfaction or quality of client outcomes. Another approach, which is less popular with accountants because it is often more costly in the short term, might be a belief system about the rights and needs of the clients, such as individualised care by a constant (often larger) team of (qualified) practitioners. Delivering client care in an environment that has strong peer support and high professional standards has a profound influence on staff job satisfaction and thus retention. Inevitably, it also promotes client satisfaction and improved outcomes, but the results are difficult to quantify and take time to be recognisable; thus they are ignored by hard-pressed senior managers with short-term targets and tight budgets to manage.

Points to ponder – formal and informal policies:
Thinking about your own workplace:

- Do you have a policy concerned with staffing levels and skill mix?
- Would you describe it as a formal or informal policy?
- Who developed this policy?
- On what basis was the policy developed (e.g., custom and practice or research evidence)?
- In what way is this policy implemented?
- What are your own views about its effect on client satisfaction and on staff satisfaction?

Policies can also influence the geographical structure of the work setting. As an example, in some health care organisations, patients have individual rooms to ensure complete privacy, but this means they cannot be seen so easily, and the level of staffing needs to be higher than when they are in a large, open space with other patients. Inevitably, the short-term staffing costs are higher. Alternatively, groups of patients may be cared for in single-sex wards to enhance supervision and reduce the need for so many staff and possibly reduce the required level of competence. This is often at the cost of personal privacy and perhaps client outcome. Other policies may be concerned with professional practice, such as client confidentiality, client safety, management of specific incidents, wearing of a uniform, lone worker, access to computerised medical results, levels of supervision and so on. The following points to ponder illustrate a simple but important example of one policy that is not often documented.

Points to ponder – policy matters:
One example of an organisational policy in health care is whether the philosophy towards its clients/patients is practised: are clients asked how they would like to be addressed (by their first name or more formally by their family name?).

- Does this take place in your own workplace?
- Is this preference documented in the patient's case notes?
- Do all members of the team adhere to this request?

- What do your answers tell you about the philosophy of your workplace, and how might it be reflected in the attitudes of staff?
- Make a note of any other examples of policies that affect the management of health care practice in your workplace.

Like the issue of how to address a client, many important practices may not be covered by any formal policy within the workplace.

Another example of an area that rarely has a clearly defined policy is the management of learners, whether they are staff or visiting learners. Most organisations require all their staff to attend statutory study sessions on key risk areas such as health and safety, fire prevention, moving and handling, but how is attendance organised and managed? And are these study days the only important kind of professional development?

Points to ponder – staff development:

- Are statutory training sessions the only type of continuing education staff experience?
- What sort of continuing education do you think should be available?
- Who do you think should pay for continuing education of individual staff, and why do you hold this view?
- Does your workplace have a formal policy to ensure that all staff have equal opportunities for continuing education?

One aspect of frustration for staff who do attend continuing education courses is that their experiences and new knowledge are ignored by the organisation. Does this happen in your organisation, or do you have a forum for feeding back new knowledge?

The support of visiting learners, is often prescribed by external professional organisations with strict criteria (defined either by the professional statutory organisation such as the Nursing and Midwifery Council or by the university) for the placement experience that includes supervisory support and a proportion of time spent under supervision. However, such policies are rarely documented in the workplace philosophy or its policies and, as a result, are often ignored by staff, which is why workloads are not reduced when practitioners are supervising a learner.

Organisation of work

Local policies can be developed that also influence the management of work. How work is organised and managed depends on the essential philosophy of the leadership and the team. Some communities of practice choose to organise their work in small teams dedicated to groups of clients, whereas others choose a system of having a named practitioner with overall responsibility for a smaller group of clients supported by a small team of staff of varying skill levels to cover each shift. Both these approaches are designed to ensure holistic care with clear lines of accountability for the quality of care, the aim being to ensure that clients receive a consistent approach to their every-day care. Learners joining the team of practitioners can also expect to receive a consistent approach to their supervision and to be able to participate in care delivery, as well as to receive feedback that is regular and frequent.

In other settings, care is delivered on a task basis according to the skill mix available. This industrial model requires a fragmentation of care and thus unclear lines of accountability for individual patients. Care is based on a hierarchy with the most sophisticated tasks such as administration of intravenous drug being undertaken by the most competent practitioner and the everyday activities delegated to the most junior staff member. Research from the 1970s and 1980s demonstrated that this approach to care delivery in nursing led to sub-standard and dehumanised care. However, for learners trying to develop expertise in specific technical skills, it does provide opportunities for consolidation of technical skills by repetitive practice.

A policy for education in the workplace

By agreeing a philosophy to inform all aspects of work, staff can develop a range of policies and protocols that in turn will promote high standards of professional practice. These include policies and protocols regarding staff development such as all staff having opportunities to receive a consistent standard of continuing education. They also govern the treatment of learners when they arrive in the placement for work experience. An essential aspect of such policies is recognition of the available resources and an aspiration that learners will leave the setting feeling encouraged and inspired by the quality of care delivered to clients and by their own personal development. With the anticipated severe shortages in professional staff owing to demographic changes, it becomes even more important that learners are encouraged to see your workplace as an attractive place to return to work on qualification. The points to ponder for valuing learning at work below illustrate a range of educational activities that practitioners can undertake informally without needing to attend formal educational sessions, study days, etc., and Chapters 9 and 10 deal with this specifically.

Points to ponder – valuing learning at work:

- Many clinical settings have an informal policy that indicates the importance of education for staff – can you summarise what the policy might be for your own workplace?
- To what extent do you and your colleagues feel part of a wider community of practice, where you maintain and further develop your professional knowledge by participating in local and national discussions, either online or through conferences and journals?

Are you and your colleagues encouraged to:

- attend and contribute to case conferences?
- initiate discussions within your own community of practice on specific topics or journal articles?
- undertake responsibility for specific and specialist aspects of the work such as prevention of infection or management of aggressive behaviour?
- join special-interest groups within the organisation, locally or nationally?

Reading through this list of developmental activities, you can see that they are not particularly time-consuming or onerous. They have the aim of helping practitioners to develop their professional knowledge, which has immediate and enduring relevance to their work. Some workplaces identify their staff as members of a community of practice, or a setting where the workers have shared professional interests, knowledge and skills. Thinking about your own workplace in this way provides you and your colleagues with opportunities to link up with like-minded practitioners to exchange ideas, discuss problems and share new initiatives and research findings. Using the internet in this manner increases opportunities for sharing best practice as well as going on exchange visits or sabbaticals to similar professional settings either nationally or internationally. Inevitably, such contacts and experiences lead to improved quality of practice. They can also provide you with new ways to support visiting learners.

Supporting visiting learners

As an established member of a team of practitioners working in a familiar setting, it is sometimes difficult to remember your own time as a learner and the challenges of starting on a new placement. With programmes of education leading to professional qualifications taking place in centralised universities or colleges, learners are frequently sent out to placements that are a considerable distance from either their homes or their education centre. Quite often, they feel very isolated unless there is an effective support structure to facilitate their placement. This is particularly true for learners going into the community for experience, and the process can be extremely stressful, as Vignette 3.1 illustrates.

Vignette 3.1   Being a newcomer – Carly's experiences

Carly is a second-year mental health nursing learner. She had worked as a part-time health care assistant for several years while her children were young. She is just finishing her placement on an acute care substance abuse unit and has found out that her next placement after her holiday is with a community psychiatric nurse (CPN) who works from a newly built medical centre, a one hour's bus journey from her home. The information that she has received so far is the name of the medical centre and that she will be posted to a CPN. Carly tries several times on different days to telephone the Medical Centre during 'normal working hours', without success. The centre does not seem to have a web address, so she cannot email anyone there. She manages to contact the mental-health learner-support nurse, Beverley, who tells her that she is expected and that she will chase up Ben (the person who is going to mentor her) and get him to text Carly with his contact details. A week before her placement is due to start, Carly has still not heard from this man, so she contacts Beverley again for help. This time, Beverley is on holiday, and there is no one else that Carly can find to help her. The medical centre is still not responding to her phone calls or messages, so she writes a letter to Ben at the centre explaining what she has done to contact him and that she understands she is due to arrive at the centre on 6 March. On 6 March, Carly gets up at 6 am to prepare her children for school and takes them to a neighbour who will look after them until it starts and then catches the 6.45 am bus to travel to the Medical Centre.

When Carly arrives at the Medical Centre, she finds it is closed, and no none is around. The notice on the door says it is not due to open until 9 am, so she goes to find a café where she can have a hot drink and some breakfast and returns at 9 am.

On her return at 9 am, she speaks to the receptionist, who does not seem to know anything about her placement and tells her that Ben has gone out on his rounds. She does, however, offer to telephone Ben on his mobile phone, which she does and hands the phone over to Carly. Ben sounds rather off-hand, complaining that he had not received any messages from Beverley or Carly's letter but will be back at the centre in an hour, and she should wait for him to return.

Question: What arrangements do you think were needed to prevent this from happening and to ensure that other learners do not suffer the same kind of experience?

Sadly, Carly's experiences might be familiar to you. Indeed, you might have had a similar experience. Most visiting learners at some time during their placement programme have been frustrated in their attempts to make arrangements for their first day or have been greeted by staff exclaiming that they were not expected, and there is no one to look after them. This is often despite the best endeavours of the manager responsible for practice education in the placements.

Most learners who are peripatetic, travelling from one work setting to another for sometimes as little as a few days or perhaps more often for a few months, worry about entering an unknown setting. They are particularly anxious to know what is expected of them, their role and responsibilities, as well as the unfamiliar technical skills they will be expected to know. Without a thoughtful and carefully planned induction period and effective support, these newcomers are likely to make mistakes as well as to have high levels of sickness or absence. It is remarkable that someone who had an experience such as Carly's (Vignette 3.1) did not give up and stay at home and wait to be called. So many learners suffer from similar acts of thoughtlessness. It is a tribute to Carly's commitment that she persisted and did take the trouble to get to her placement at the time required.

It is also so easy to prevent situations like Carly's, with a bit of thought, preparation and communication, which will be of benefit to clients and staff, as well as to learners. This preparation is best undertaken according to an informal or formal agreement, preferably as a documented policy that all staff know about and support. Such a policy tells visiting learners what kinds of educational and developmental support they can expect from your work setting. Box 3.1 contains some suggestions for preparing a policy for your visiting learners for their placement.

Much of the information outlined in Box 3.1 may be already available to learners coming to your workplace online, through your own organisation's intranet web site or in paper form. Many workplaces have a member of staff who is identified as being responsible

---

Box 3.1 Supporting visiting learners: a framework.

- Information about the workplace: its aims and the client group that it serves; working hours, meal-break times, dress code, travel considerations; location of policies and protocols; contact details
- Key staff members and those staff who are qualified to offer supervision
- Other visiting learners who may be present in the setting at any time
- Learning experiences in the setting, for example, attendance at case conferences, specific therapies provided, activities or workshops used by clients;
- External learning experiences associated with the clients' overall care pathway, for example, visits to associated relevant departments such as outpatient department, investigatory departments, treatment clinics, home visits with professional colleagues
- Guidance on what preparation the visiting learner needs to undertake prior to starting in the setting
- Supervision arrangements: name and contact details of designated supervisor and normal supervising arrangements, including sharing shift times
- Orientation programme: what it will cover and how soon into the placement it will take place
- Assessment of learner capability: a strategy used to ensure client safety is maintained and to allow planning to meet each learner's developmental needs

for professional education and for supporting visiting learners. This person has the task of ensuring that everyone in the workplace also knows what they can and should be offering to visiting learners as well as to ensure that the policy is up to date and is known by all the staff. Making this kind of information available on the intranet helps visiting learners to access the material quickly and easily. The team can use this kind of information to promote their good practices and to both reassure and stimulate enquiry and learning. Information like this offers reassurance, as it provides learners with essential information while implying a welcoming commitment by the team to supporting learners. It helps learners to plan their attendance: how to find the venue, who to contact, what to wear and so on. It also tells them what to expect. Such information can be stimulating, as it provides newcomers with a sense of responsibility for their own learning in an environment that is evidently committed to supporting education and good practice, as Vignette 3.2 illustrates. A good web page with helpful information can also help with recruiting new staff.

Vignette 3.2   Welcome to our team!

Anya is a 20-year-old radiography learner and is about to start her first placement in a large teaching hospital 5 miles from her university and her rooms. The placement is for 12 weeks. She has been in contact with the clinical teacher for the hospital who has given her access to the hospital intranet web site and advised Anya to look at the radiography unit site. On their site, she finds a special web page dedicated to visiting learners, outlining the working hours, the different sections of the unit and their specialisms. It also includes a page with the photographs of all the members of staff along with their professional qualifications, making it easy for Anya to recognise them. There is a section with advice about starting on the unit as well as some information sheets and interactive 'workbooks' that she can download to help her learn about the techniques she will be encountering. She even finds a hyperlink to a Facebook page of the person she is going to have as her supervisor, so that she can start communicating with her straight away. Through their Facebook chat, they arrange a time for Anya to start on the unit as well as a meeting point.

Questions: How do you think Anya felt about starting her placement on this unit? What do arrangements such as these tell you about this unit as a place to work and to learn? Does your workplace have similar arrangements? How possible might it be to create them?

This section of the chapter has explored the important factors that influence a workplace and the quality of the learning experiences that it offers its staff and visiting learners. Where there is a good learning environment, the quality of practice is often of a high standard as well. Explanations are usually influenced by the social environment, such as: the quality of leadership and style of management, existence of a team spirit, a commitment to personal and colleague development; a commitment to delivering high standards of evidence-based practice; a commitment to ensuring best practice for the client; and a desire to communicate best practice to learners. Inevitably, there are other factors that facilitate such an environment, including: the overall philosophy and management of the organisation as a whole and its commitment to its staff and to its clients; and the efficient and effective management of resources, effective communication at all levels of the organisation.

One strategy that helps practitioners to provide high standards of work and to achieve the organisational aims is the development of protocols. A protocol is a 'user guide' to a specific activity, and it is most effective when developed from an evidence base.

Protocols

Protocols are normally prescriptions for practice designed to ensure a consistent and high standard of practice. They are developed from research or evidence-based practice and intended to support practitioners unfamiliar with a specific health care condition or where care is delivered mostly by non-professionally qualified staff. They provide invaluable support to learners and to newly qualified staff working in unfamiliar settings, and they promote a consistent approach to practice. Sometimes, newcomers discover that the clinical setting uses different, 'unauthorised' protocols, and often they have been decreed by a senior member of the team, usually the consultant medical practitioner. Visiting learners, particularly, struggle to cope with informal practices when they see that accepted protocols are being undermined by local practice, as a nursing learner discovered in Vignette 3.3:

Vignette 3.3   Using evidence-based practice

Gavin is a second-year nursing learner and has started working on a surgical ward. He is keen to develop his skills in giving intramuscular injections. He has had practical preparation in the Skills Laboratory at university and has read the research papers about preparation of the skin. He is working with his mentor, Minna, an experienced registered nurse, and during the morning shift, they prepare patients for surgery, with Gavin giving the intramuscular injections. By lunchtime, he is feeling more confident in giving injections. His mentor then goes off-duty, so in the afternoon he is supervised by a different nurse, Frances. When a patient needs intramuscular pain relief, Gavin tells Frances that he would like to carry on practising this technique, however, in the process of giving the injection, Frances tells him off for not preparing the skin appropriately. Gavin is quite shocked, as he knows he has been following the correct protocol. So, what has happened?

It seems that Frances either has not maintained her professional knowledge or is following an informal protocol for giving injections. Sadly, her actions have wrecked Gavin's new-found confidence as well as his trust in Frances.

This vignette illustrates how learners can be confused by a slight difference in professional practice. It is unlikely that there is a written protocol to cover this taken-for-granted procedure, so it is easy for someone like Frances, who has been using her technique for many years, not to have realised that she needed to update her knowledge; whereas her colleague, Minna, does know about the recent changes, perhaps because of her own professional development or because she let a visiting learner share her knowledge. In this situation, the patient does not come to any harm, but it can cause a great deal of psychological harm to a learner who is already lacking in confidence and assuming clinical staff to be conforming to best-practice guidelines.

In large organisations, there are often a range of practices that contravene evidence-based protocols or protocols designed to protect confidentiality. Sometimes, such protocols have a counter-productive effect such as strict rules about access to computerised information. Limiting access to confidential information to certain members of staff is obviously sensible except in some regularly occurring situations such as staff changeover. New staff such as newly appointed medical officers starting at a weekend or before a formal induction period are unable to function unless they can get access to computerised results from investigative procedures. They may even find access to departments out of hours impossible because of security procedures owing to 'common-sense' protocols (Kilminster et al. 2010: 565). As a result, staff have to find ways of navigating around the protocol in order to do their job. Other, perhaps more important, protocols that are often disregarded are concerned with client care, such as: poor or absent management of patient mobility and independence; lack of use of reality-orientation strategies when caring for confused or hallucinating patients; and inappropriate drug prescription and administration. Protocols relating to these and many other essential health care practices can make a huge difference to patient recovery.

Policies and protocols are the organisational standards that every member of the organisation is expected to adhere to. However, in every setting, there are a range of informal, unwritten protocols that only people who have been working in the setting for some time are familiar with. More often than not, these informal protocols are the ones that are observed by staff the most rigorously. A newcomer to the setting will not know about them until they have been working in the setting for some time, unless they have a friendly advisor or a supervisor who is aware of such protocols and can fully orientate them to the setting. Many visiting learners and newcomers entering an unfamiliar workplace find that their education and knowledge are undermined by local practices, such as the experiences of Annah (Snapshot 3.1), a new member of the registered nursing staff who has been working overseas for several years for an aid organisation. Following an orientation period within the Trust, she has now started working in the Accident and Emergency Department (A&E).

Snapshot 3.1   Annah, protocols and everyday practice

This is Annah's third week in the A&E Department, and she is on night duty. It is a typically hectic Saturday night. A group of very drunk teenagers arrive at midnight with a friend who has severe bruises and lacerations to his face and upper torso, some of which look more like stab wounds. Annah calls the doctor to inspect the wounds, but he is very busy elsewhere in the department and unlikely to be free for at least 2 h. Annah examines the boy fully to assess his condition (including a neurological assessment) and the extent of any blood loss. She takes photographs of the wounds and documents his account of what happened. With the boy's consent, she contacts the police officer who is on duty in the Department and tells him what the boy has told her. Annah takes a blood sample for tests as well as group- and cross-matching. Because her observations suggest he is dehydrated, Annah sets up a slow intravenous infusion of dextrose–saline and then swabs the wounds for infection before dressing and suturing them. She arranges for him to have a skull and chest X-ray, in case he has any fractures. It is now 2 h since the boy arrived in A&E, and the doctor has still not arrived, despite Annah's requests for assistance from him. Annah then administers anti-tetanus intramuscularly. She feels he needs intravenous antibiotics and analgesia, but in view of her assessment of his neurological condition and without a medical prescription, she cannot give the drugs. All of Annah's actions comply with the normal protocols for such incidents, except they are normally initiated and conducted by the on-duty doctor.

At 4 am, the doctor arrives to see the boy and is shocked to see the extent of Annah's actions. He tells Annah that he will be making a formal complaint about her actions to the Unit manager. Annah is bewildered and upset by this reaction. In the past, she has had extensive experience of working in similar situations and is a highly competent critical care nurse. She is also quite convinced that her actions have saved the boy's life.

Points to ponder:

Annah has had extensive experience in this field of practice and is highly competent in delivering this kind of care. However, the Trust policy does not permit nurses to undertake such an extended role without undergoing an approved training programme (which Annah has not yet taken)

- Do you think it is reasonable for Annah to have carried out the actions that she did?
- What actions do you think the Trust management will take following the doctor's complaint?
- Where are such policies and protocols documented and stored in your organisation?
- How are new staff to your workplace orientated to policies concerning role, and extended role? (i.e., Who tells the new member of staff? When are they told? Is this induction information documented anywhere?)

In Snapshot 3.1, Annah was fulfilling a familiar role in a time of crisis for the Department and as a result may face a disciplinary hearing. In Vignette 3.3, Gavin is confused by variations in delivery of a technical skill, and while the variations are not critical, they are the result of increased research and understanding. Both these situations illustrate dilemmas where local practices contradict protocols and perhaps common sense. Such contradictions can be very confusing for newcomers and peripatetic learners. Sometimes, informal protocols are developed as a means of 'getting by' with limited resources, or by coming to different conclusions from the research or occasionally as a result of ignorance. Whatever the situation, it is worth while developing strategies to ensure that staff are aware of these nuances and that new staff and visiting learners also need to be made aware of them (Kilminster et al. 2011).

Point to ponder – formal and informal protocols:

Think of at least two informal policies/practices that influence your approach to work. They could be the preferences of the senior manager or clinician, or 'how things are always done':

- Why do you think these informal protocols are developed?
- How does a newcomer find out about these informal policies/practices in your own setting?
- How can you reassure a learner that this informal protocol is a legitimate approach?

Collaborative learning among the professions

In Chapter 4, we will be discussing the micro aspects of the learning environment, the inter-personal aspects. An important aspect of this micro environment is provision of opportunities for learners to work with, and to learn from, other professionals. Government and professional policies have long advocated that learners should spend much of their programme working and learning together, the aim being to increase understanding of each other's role, the issues they face and how collaboration can be achieved to improve the patient/client experience. Creating structures within pre-qualification educational programmes to achieve these aims has proved incredibly difficult, essentially because sharing a common curriculum is often complicated by competing professional requirements. Placements provide the most attractive solution to the challenge of inter-professional learning and working. Most placements have either permanent or visiting staff from a range of professions and so are ideal settings to afford their visiting learners (and staff) opportunities to have practical experiences of each other's role. Establishing this kind of provision is a policy that every placement needs to establish as an essential so that all its members of staff consider it to be a natural part of their work. Vignette 3.4a provides an example of inter-professional opportunities.

Vignette 3.4a   Working and learning together

Malangan is an oncology unit in a regional cancer centre. It welcomes a range of learners on a regular basis. After a great deal of discussion with eight different professional programme representatives from the university (social work, complementary therapies, nutritional therapy, radiotherapy, nursing, medicine, occupational therapy and medical scientists), a policy was agreed, and a protocol was developed that described what visiting learners must achieve during their placement. This included:

- development of a comprehensive care pathway plan demonstrating consideration of the range of support and treatment services available;
- presentation of the plan to peers and associated professionals at an end-of-placement conference;
- documentation of the finalised care pathway plan with rationale for each aspect, as an assignment for the end-of-module assessment.

The policy ensured that all members of the unit were conversant with the programme learners were undertaking and were willing to support the learners. The protocol provided guidelines for the supervisors and their learners. It also meant that resources were developed and made available for the learners to use.

It is quite possible that learners from different professions come to your workplace at different times. This does not negate the importance of ensuring they have opportunities to learn from other professional colleagues; it just means that your policy and protocols need to be designed to reflect what is achievable within your setting. Vignette 3.4b provides an alternative example:

Vignette 3.4b   Working and learning together

Rivendale is a rural general practice unit serving a community of 40 000 people. It is staffed by four medical practitioners, two practice nurses, a pharmacist, a diabetic specialist, three community nurses, two community care assistants, a social worker and a psychotherapist. The practice manager and her team of administrative staff run the practice. The Practice is also supported by a team of community midwives, two health visitors and a community physiotherapist, based in the town some 3 miles away. They come into the practice on a regular basis. The midwives conduct antenatal and post-natal assessments, and the health visitors offer weekly health checks on babies and toddlers as well as for the older residents registered with the practice. Once a month, a nutritionist and the diabetic specialist hold a clinic to advise service users on how to manage their diet or to eat healthily. The physiotherapist has two clinics a week to give rehabilitation therapy for a range of patients. A phlebotomist and laboratory technician visit the centre once a week for patients needing regular blood tests.

Following consultation with the Practice Board members, the community inter-professional facilitator has established a programme for all learners who visit the practice. This programme includes attending clinics, going out on visits with the different professionals and writing a profile of the Practice and the community it serves, which includes recommendations for future health and social care services.

You can appreciate that learners attending Rivendale Practice unit can have a rich experience of health and social care provision in the community. The wide range of professionals that work in association with the Practice affords exposure to their work as well as to the everyday health needs of the residents. By requiring learners to document their experiences and to develop judgements, they have to apply their learning in a more profound and meaningful way that is more memorable. As a result, learners have the opportunity to develop a deep understanding of how professionals can work together to the benefit of the community.

Summary

A workplace that is unfamiliar to newcomers presents a number of challenges. This chapter illustrates how the quality of a learning environment depends upon a range of organisational and human factors. Perhaps the two most important factors are concerned with the quality of leadership and the attitude of staff. If these people have a commitment to high standards of practice and to promoting professional development, they are more likely to ensure that visiting learners are prepared for work in the setting, and they are supported effectively while they are there.

Working in a community of practice where each practitioner feels established and confident in their role provides a satisfying place to work and increases the satisfaction of the clients/patients.

Appendix 3.1 Audit tool for the placement learning environment.

	Strongly agree	Agree	Disagree	Strongly disagree
Physical aspects of the learning environment Geography – is your workplace a compact and discrete environment, or is it spread over a wide geographical area? Is the area adequate for the function of the team? Are the facilities appropriate for the client group at all stages of their care? Are there adequate storage facilities for the resources, and is access to them appropriate? Is communication between staff facilitated by the physical resources, for example, internet access, handheld systems? Are there places where staff can meet each other both formally and informally? Can equipment or other resources be ordered and delivered effectively and on time?				
Social aspects of the learning environment Staffing: is it adequate and of the correct skill mix for the work of the setting, including the number of peripatetic learners, for example, do professional staff undertake clerical work in the absence of a clerk or vice versa? Does the skill mix account for the increased workload of learner supervision? Are there structures in place to ensure staff meet regularly and frequently for peer support, and for exchange of information, for problem-solving? Is the quality of communication effective between internal staff and senior management of the institution and with visiting staff? Is there effective leadership within the clinical team? Are the relationships between the different professional groups associated with the work focus effective and constructive? Is there effective management of the team? Are there effective structures to ensure policies and protocols are implemented? Do staff have clear and effective guidelines and avenues of management when dealing with difficult and challenging situations?				

(continued)

Appendix 3.1   *(cont'd)*

	Strongly agree	Agree	Disagree	Strongly disagree
Professional aspects of the learning environment				
Are the purpose and the function of the workplace clear and respected?				
Are the staffing and skill mix appropriate for the nature of clients?				
Are staff adequately and appropriately prepared for the nature of work and for the clients?				
Are staff appropriately prepared to support learners?				
Is the breadth of professional support appropriate for the client group, that is, are the appropriate clinical specialists available to provide advice and support to the clients and the staff?				
Are protocols and professional practices implemented to the highest standards, and are these audited on a regular and frequent basis?				
Are continuing education and use of evidence-based practices promoted and implemented?				
Are the equipment and other resources appropriate for the nature of work?				
Are visiting learners encouraged to participate fully in the work of the team based on their assessed capability?				
Are learners encouraged to participate in case conferences and team meetings?				
Is there effective communication between the setting and the educational providers and their local representatives?				
Are there regular visits from other members of the health and social care team to support the client care package?				
Are support services effective?				
Philosophical and educational aspects of the learning environment				
Is there a mission statement, or statement of beliefs, agreed and documented that informs the work of the team?				
Is there evidence that the mission statement influences all aspects of practice?				
Is work allocated on the basis of capability and as a means of supervised professional development?				
Are clients' wishes identified and respected?				

Appendix 3.1   *(cont'd)*

	Strongly agree	Agree	Disagree	Strongly disagree
Are clients treated according to the highest of professional standards?				
Are clients and their carers invited to evaluate their care?				
Is staff education an important and continuous part of the overall function of the team?				
Are staff encouraged to implement new practices and thinking?				
Is there an agreement about the number, range and skill mix of visiting learners?				
Does the range of visiting learners reflect the available skill mix to ensure their adequate support and supervision?				
Are there effective policies on the support and supervision of visiting learners?				
Is staff workload adjusted when supervising a learner?				
Is learner feedback encouraged and acted upon?				
Are there written guidelines and documented learning opportunities for visiting learners made available to them prior to arrival?				
Are there planned opportunities for learners from different professions to work or learn alongside each other?				

Chapter 4

Practice settings as a learning resource

Jenny Spouse

Introduction

In Chapter 3, we looked at the workplace as a learning environment from the perspective of internal organisational and local policies and protocols, and how they influence the way a workplace functions. In this chapter, we explore how professional policies influence the structure of a professional programme and how the workplace can be an important source of professional development and education.

Visiting learners will have been allocated to your specific workplace because of what it has to offer and because of requirements from their professional statutory organisation. Many of these requirements are determined by government and professional policies influenced by predictions of future health care or social service delivery needs, which in turn are influenced by demographic changes and the health of the population. Another important influence are requirements of the European Commission, partly designed to facilitate population movement within its borders by ensuring equivalency of professional qualifications between its member states. These policies subsequently influence the professional statutory organisations who stipulate the content of professional programmes.

Placements for pre-qualification learners are normally agreed after extensive consultation between funding agencies of the government, the service providers (community and institutional agencies) and the educational providers (higher or further education organisations). Instrumental to the success of a placement as a learning environment is the ability of the resident practitioners to promote learning.

The emphasis in this chapter is to take a long view on how practice may be considered as an educational experience and to develop a curriculum from which newcomers and visiting learners can negotiate a learning plan for their own learning according to their professional needs. The chapter will include some suggestions for you to explore the resources that you and your colleagues might use to promote learning and to develop a learning curriculum.

This chapter includes the following:

- external influences on professional education from national and international policies; commissioning professional programmes;
- collaborative curriculum design;

Practice-Based Learning in Nursing, Health and Social Care: Mentorship, Facilitation and Supervision,
First Edition. Ian Scott and Jenny Spouse.

- curriculum planning for placements;
- creating a curriculum for practice – practice as knowledge; developing learning resources and making them accessible;
- quality assurance.

External influences on professional education

Professional education is influenced by globalisation. Across the world, many health and social care practitioners work alongside professional colleagues from different parts of the world, whose qualifications are recognised by their professional statutory regulatory organisation. Facilitating this inter-state migration is recognition of the equivalency of qualifications. To achieve this, the World Health Organization (WHO) has led inter-state discussions leading to agreement on the structure and content of professional preparatory programmes. The WHO aims to improve the status of (health care) practitioners across the world and to set consistent international standards for their preparation. In Europe, the WHO framework has been used by the European Commission to create its own directives affecting the preparation of architects, dentists, doctors, 'general' nurses, midwives, pharmacists and vetinary surgeons, again to ensure equivalence of qualifications, thus promoting cross-border mobility and employment within the European community. Two Articles from the European Union Directives for 'general nurses', outlined in Box 4.1 Articles 3 & 5 of the European Union, prescribe the length of the programme, who has responsibility for its provision, responsibility for the teaching of learners, and the experiences learners must be afforded. It is an example of how international organisations influence national policies on professional education.

Box 4.1   Articles 3 & 5 of the European Union Standards for Nursing and Midwifery Education (European Union 2005).

Article 3:

The training of nurses responsible for general care shall comprise at least three years of study or 4600 hours of theoretical and clinical training, the duration of the theoretical training representing at least one-third and the duration of the clinical training at least one-half of the minimum duration of the training.

Article 5:

Clinical training is that part of nurse training in which trainee nurses learn, as part of a team and in direct contact with a healthy or sick individual and/or community, to organize, dispense and evaluate the required comprehensive nursing care, on the basis of the knowledge and skills which they have acquired. The trainee nurse shall learn not only how to work in a team, but also how to lead a team and organize overall nursing care, including health education for individuals and small groups, within the health institute or in the community. This training shall take place in hospitals and other health institutions and in the community, under the responsibility of nursing teachers, in cooperation with and assisted by other qualified nurses. Other qualified personnel may also take part in the teaching process.

---

http://eur-lex.europa.eu, © European Union, 1998–2012.

Points to ponder:

- What are your views of these articles?
- Reading through these articles, how do they compare with the requirements of your own professional statutory regulatory organisation?
- Can you identify any aspects of your own professional preparation that may have been influenced by these directives from the European Union?
- Can you think of any other international influences on your professional training programme?

The requirements of the European Union identified in Box 4.1 are normally agreed as a result of collaboration between representatives of the member governments and their professional statutory organisations. Detailed discussion of national provision for professional education often results from widespread consultations with the public, registrants or members, and associated agencies such as the Royal Colleges in the United Kingdom. In addition, research reports and studies are commissioned to advise these Colleges so that they can make provision for future populations. An example of a nursing education consultation is the paper commissioned by the Nursing and Midwifery Council of the United Kingdom, 'Nursing Towards 2015', which identified 12 paradoxes in health care (see Table 4.1) to illustrate the challenges when planning for the future.

Table 4.1   Paradoxes of future health care in the United Kingdom.

1	Availability of funding	And	Unequal distribution and need
2	Regional disparities	And	Shared constraints
3	Priority given to preventative measures	And	Expectation of cure and palliative care
4	Hospitals as the dominant provider	And	Policy to deliver care in the community
5	Drive for increased technology	And	Public appetite for alternative therapies
6	Influence of professionals	And	Increased assertiveness by the public
7	More well-educated, informed and confident consumers	And	Many patients who lack information and confidence
8	Nurses need to be competent in new technologies and to be problem solvers	And	Value of humanistic approaches and the time they require
9	Blurring of professional boundaries	And	Entrenched distinctiveness of professions and public expectations
10	Changing demography of health and illness	And	Changing fashions in health care provision and expectations
11	Moral certainties valued	And	New technologies creating ethical dilemmas and uncertainty
12	Public expectations of nurses	And	Nurses' expectations to assume new roles and responsibilities

Adapted from: Longley, Shaw & Dolan 2007 'Nursing: Towards 2015'.

Navigating an acceptable solution to these identified paradoxes and the complexity of preparing practitioners for the future is challenging and uncertain. One of the most enduring and difficult aspects of designing new rules for new programmes is the availability of adequate funds to implement the solution. Education is expensive, and professional education even more so, because of the potential risk to the public and the need for a range of educators to supervise learners. More often than not, governments avoid committing themselves to full funding of these programmes, hence the reliance on resident practitioners to supervise learners in the workplace. This supervision often is provided without extra funding or extra staff.

Commissioning and developing professional programmes

Professional programmes are normally commissioned on behalf of the funding agency (the government) by local workforce planning agencies. Their aim is to ensure a continuous supply of suitably prepared practitioners based on anticipated changes in the workforce. To inform their planning, commissioners use data on future staffing needs, resulting from retirement numbers, staff turnover and staff requirements for planned developments, such as closure of hospitals and increased reliance on community services. So, for example, if there is a policy to deliver more care in the community to mental-health patients, the structure of the workforce needs to reflect this policy change, with recruitment of more social workers, more community mental-health nurses and more community rehabilitation facilities. Commissioners may decide that a range of post-qualification programmes are required to prepare current practitioners. They may also decide that pre-qualification programmes need to have a stronger emphasis on care in the community and that health care providers need to offer more placements for learners to facilitate this, leaving it to local managers to ensure they have sufficient staff to supervise the extra learners.

Adult Education Institutions (AEIs) compete and negotiate to receive these commissions with strictly defined funding to recruit specific numbers of learners to specific programmes. Out of this funding comes the cost of staff salaries, structural costs such as use of classrooms and resources, and any staff development costs. The ability of an AEI to provide the commissioned courses is often restricted by the range of local health and social care providers, and thus the placement experiences available to support the curriculum, particularly of pre-qualification programmes. Post-qualification programme provision is similarly affected. For example, if the commissioning agents decide that they should fund a National Health Service regional centre for cardiac surgery, it will need to ensure there are sufficient suitably qualified personnel to staff the unit and to support the patients throughout their health care pathway. This will be a complex team including diagnostic, technical, laboratory, medical, nursing, physio-therapy, social work staff, as well as others. To be successful and to ensure the continuity of staffing, the centre will have to provide training facilities for learners from all the associated professions, which means they will need supervision and a local adult education institution able to offer educational programmes. When planning for this kind of programme, placements are normally audited to identify the range of clinical learning opportunities available. As you may appreciate, planning a curriculum and negotiating access for learners to placements from a wide geographical area and across a range of service providers is a complex process.

Collaborative curriculum design

You will recognise from these earlier paragraphs that planning and delivering a professional programme to prepare learners for their professional qualification is subject to policies and directives issues by a range of organisations: the World Health Organisation, the European

Union, the (UK) government, the professional statutory regulatory organisation, the local commissioners and the local health care providers.

A curriculum planning team is normally made up of representatives from the local health and social care providers, and representatives from the educational team delivering the programme. Together, they agree the philosophy of the programme, and its overall aims and objectives. For example, the planning team has to address questions such as:

- To what extent will the qualification be generic?
- Will learners exit the programme with specialist qualifications to meet the needs of specific client groups, such as mental health, care of older people, etc.?
- Can people with subsidiary professional qualifications step on to the programme at specified points?
- Can learners step off the programme with a lesser qualification?
- How long should the course take?
- Should full-time health/social care learners have time off from their programme during the vacation periods as for other higher-education learners, thus denying them the opportunity to earn?

Questions such as these are also influenced by continuing discussions among and within professional organisations and the funding agencies. Local policies often influence the nature of the qualification that learners have on completion of their pre-qualification programme. In the United Kingdom, the majority of nurses preparing for the professional Register are trained to nurse adult patients. With demographic and policy changes, an increasing proportion of graduates are needed to work in the community rather than in a hospital. So, will a curriculum that is dominated traditionally by hospital placements be suitable for nurses who will ultimately work in the community? Or should they have a separate and possibly overlapping curriculum that may limit their flexibility for future employment options? Similar dilemmas face programme planners for other professions such as occupational therapy (OT) and social work. Should learners be given a generic programme with post-qualification study in the specialist area, or should programmes provide different avenues for specialist practice such as OT work in industrial settings, or with older people or those in rehabilitation?

With government policies requiring all professional programmes to include opportunities to learn and work alongside learners from other professions, how much of the programme can be inter-professional, that is, will learners from the different professions take classes in the AEI together, and if so, which classes? Which placements can offer inter-professional experiences, and how should these be managed? Planning to manage details of these kinds is fraught with complexity, as are decisions about where learners may be placed for their practical experiences, and at what stage of their programme. In nursing, some of these decisions are forced upon the curriculum planners by the EU requirements (see Table 4.2).

In defining the nature of clinical instruction, the European Union stated that 'It is the part of the programme where nursing learners are supervised while in direct contact with healthy and sick individuals or communities, to learn to plan, provide and assess the required total nursing care on the basis of their acquired knowledge and skills'.

These directives require the learner nurse not only to be a member of a team, but also to be a team leader organising total nursing care, including health education for individuals and small groups in health institutions or the community.

Table 4.2 European Union requirements of adult (general) nursing programmes.

Article 5.2.1. Training programme for nurses responsible for general care		
The training leading to the award of a formal qualification of nurses responsible for general care shall consist of the following two parts.		
A. Theoretical instruction including: i. Nursing: ii. Basic sciences: iii. Social sciences:		**B. Clinical instruction: Nursing in relation to:**
Nature and ethics of the profession General principles of health and nursing Nursing principles in relation to: General and specialist medicine General and specialist surgery Child care and paediatrics Maternity care Mental health and psychiatry Care of the old and geriatrics Principles of administration Social and health legislation	Anatomy and physiology Pathology Bacteriology, virology and parasitology Biophysics, biochemistry and radiology Dietetics Hygiene Preventive medicine Health education Pharmacology Sociology Psychology Principles of teaching Legal aspects of nursing	General and specialist medicine General and specialist surgery Child care and paediatrics Maternity care Mental health and psychiatry Care of the old and geriatrics Home nursing One or more of these subjects may be taught in the context of the other disciplines or in conjunction therewith
The theoretical instruction must be weighted and coordinated with the clinical instruction in such a way that the knowledge and skills referred to in this Annex can be acquired in an adequate fashion.		

European Standards for Nursing and Midwifery Education (2004), WHO.

In the United Kingdom, this definition from the European Union provides the framework prescribed by the Nursing and Midwifery Council (NMC) known as the Proficiencies. Achievement of which is required of all candidates applying for professional registration. In 2011, the NMC updated their Standards for curriculum design by reaffirming that nursing is a practice-based profession and that respect and the well-being of the patients and clients are the core focus (Nursing and Midwifery Council of the United Kingdom 2012). In arguing that entry to the nursing register should become all-graduate, the NMC identifies five principles that are enshrined in the following:

- the NMC code of professional conduct: standards for conduct, performance and ethics applies to all aspects of practice;
- nursing is an evidence-based profession;
- life-long learning and continuing professional development are valued;
- skills and knowledge are transferable;
- learners are actively involved in care delivery under supervision.

From these statements about nursing education, you can appreciate the constraints under which a curriculum planning team will be working and the requirements that must be incorporated into the programme.

Points to ponder – your professional regulatory requirements:
You have been reading about the international and national influences on adult education institutions to structure their pre-qualifying 'general' nursing programmes. To what extent does your own profession experience these kinds of influences when designing a pre-qualification programme?

Curriculum planning for placements

When planning a curriculum for placement experiences, the person responsible for the programme in the Adult Education Institution that prepares learners may establish several small working groups made up of representatives from different professional specialities. These working groups decide on the content of a specific theme in the programme and how learners can obtain the professional practical experience needed to meet regulatory requirements. The working group also must ensure learners have sufficient time in the identified placements to develop the necessary knowledge and that the throughput, that is, the number of learners at any one time and the duration of their allocation to the placement, is manageable. Decisions like this are imprecise and based on complex considerations as illustrated in Table 4.3.

Table 4.3 Considerations when placing learners.

Curriculum issues	Placement issues
Overall number of learners to be placed	Number of suitable placements
Minimum/maximum length of placement	Number of learners each placement can accommodate
Number of learners to each placement	Stage in programme learners can be accommodated (i.e., junior/intermediate/
Number of learners at same/different stage in programme attending placement at any one time	senior)
Knowledge to be gained from placement	Core/generic skills available
	Opportunities to meet professional statutory requirements
Time in the programme for placement	Specific skills available and relevance to the curriculum
More than one placement in specialist area?	Number of staff with suitable teaching skills and experience

Table 4.3 shows some of the different considerations that need to be made when planning a cycle of placements that match the professional requirements and thus influence the overall structure of the curriculum. It illustrates the impossibility of ensuring that each learner has exactly the same experiences during their overall programme.

Decisions about the numbers and 'skill mix' of learners entering a placement depend upon factors such as:

- the number and skill mix of staff available to support learners;
- the range of experience available (number of clients/patients and their health or social care needs);
- the range of other health or social care professionals that learners could be exposed to, that is, shared or inter-professional learning opportunities available.

Planning decisions may also be influenced by professional requirements and whether learners need to have several opportunities to develop the same range of skills in different but similar settings. Alternatively, the curriculum-planning team may decide that fewer but longer placements are better. For example, a learner preparing for registration in the field of learning disabilities will need experiences of working with people in their homes as well as in sheltered accommodation and in a range of relevant support agencies. It may be appropriate for the learner to be exposed to such experiences several times in different settings or to have longer placements during their two- or three-year programme. As learners increase in competence, their ability and need to gain more sophisticated kinds of professional knowledge develop, and so it is debatable whether they are more likely to profit from longer but fewer placements or vice versa.

The intention of designing placements is to facilitate learners to develop their professional knowledge and skills to the required standard for qualification and, subsequently, for autonomous practice. Inevitably, when there are a limited number of placements and a large number of learners, compromises have to be made, while ensuring the professional standards are met. Streaming learners through highly specialist areas, such as a maternity delivery suite or an intensive-care unit, poses a number of difficult challenges. In adult (general) nursing, for example, learners are required to have experience of maternity care, so what kind of experience should they have? If a large number of nursing learners are constantly passing through the delivery suit for maybe one or two days each in order to satisfy the EU requirements, what are the implications for other learners with greater statutory and educational needs, such as midwifery and medical learners? What are the implications for the permanent staff? Perhaps there are alternative placements where learners can meet the EU and professional requirements without putting such a strain on limited resources, such as in the community. So, it may be possible to reduce such a strain on the placement staff and enhance the learning experience for all learners by creative thinking and interpretation of the requirements.

When there are a small number of learners commissioned to take a programme and a large number of suitable placements, deciding where learners should have their practical experiences is relatively easy. Inevitably, when the converse is true, national and local policies also militate against ensuring adequate learner experience and support. An example from pre-registration nursing education is where the majority of placements are within hospitals. The professional statutory organisation requires learner supervision to be from a registered and 'suitably' trained professional. Local policies tend to employ unqualified staff to work as care assistants with few registered nurses to manage the wards and departments. In addition, national policies are aimed at reducing the number of hospitals and increasing care in the community. Somewhere between the requirements of the profession and policies made by government and local agencies, learners have to receive supervised and appropriate practical experience of a high standard and be assessed for their suitability for professional registration by a registered practitioner.

For programme providers to respond to the different pressures from national and local policy makers and to deliver programmes that meet professional requirements, lateral thinking and a range of compromises are required. Often this is reflected in the (generic) learning outcomes that have to be achieved during each placement and which have to be interpreted and applied to the specific context of the placement by clinical staff on the 'floor'. This is where having a curriculum for practice and a learning agenda for your visiting learners becomes an essential tool for promoting your own workplace as an effective learning environment while helping them to meet the professional requirements of their course.

Creating a curriculum for practice and a learning agenda

Few practitioners working in practice settings appreciate the wealth of knowledge that they have at their finger tips. Some researchers call this professional 'craft knowledge' or 'finger tip' knowledge, as it has become mostly intuitive. Craft knowledge is often difficult for practitioners to talk about, especially to newcomers or learners who may not share the same vocabulary. Such knowledge is concerned not only with everyday interpersonal and technical activities but also with knowledge about what happens to clients at different points in their health care pathway and the preparation or support that they are likely to need. Craft knowledge is also about knowing how to contact the appropriate person when needing advice or support and knowing the different roles of colleagues within the organisation, including associated professionals, as well as much more. Documenting this goldmine of knowledge is an important way to ensure newcomers and visiting learners can access such knowledge. One way is to develop a menu of experiences and the learning that is available in your placement. A formal term for such a menu is a curriculum.

Developing a practice-based learning curriculum is essentially a very simple task. It is a list of all the different kinds of activities that occur in your workplace and which a newcomer who is unfamiliar with the work will need to learn in order to function effectively. A study by Edmond (2001) in a Scottish hospital found that new nursing staff stayed longer, and turnover dropped, while the quality of care improved when existing staff were able to describe and document the special nature of their work. This was because they (the old timers) had been able to articulate their knowledge and to document it as well as to describe it to help newcomers quickly gain the necessary knowledge to function effectively in the setting. Depending upon their level of experience, most newly appointed staff arrive in the workplace with a degree of self-confidence and knowledge of what they will be experiencing. The same is rarely true for pre-qualification learners, who are unlikely to have any prior experience of the kind of work practised in the setting. Visiting learners are also entering the workplace with specific course objectives to be achieved during their placement, and their future career depends on their success in achieving them.

During the course curriculum planning, your workplace will have been identified as suitable for learners because of the special knowledge and skills it can help them to develop. However, this information is not always explicit to visiting learners or, as Edmond (2001) discovered, indeed to the team of staff working in the setting. When the workplace team have developed and agreed a curriculum of learning experiences, they need to make it available to learners. This puts their professional knowledge into a 'concrete' or public form that makes it more accessible. When visiting learners are given access to such a curriculum, it enables them to take a mature approach to their learning and to negotiate a structure to their placement experience. Table 4.4 provides an example of some of the learning experiences available to visiting learners in a unit specialising in the acute phase of rehabilitating people following a serious physical or neurological injury, and which has been developed in consultation with all members of the multi-disciplinary team.

Table 4.4 Curriculum of learning opportunities at Rothermead rehabilitation unit.

Generic experiences	Profession-specific experiences
Attend ward rounds and case conferences, weekly inter-professional tutorials Participate during visits to: physiotherapy unit, rehabilitation activities; occupational therapy unit including discharge preparation; clients' homes for assessment and planning of modifications necessary; accompany residents for social outings and activities; attend sessions with the social worker to appreciate the role and how clients may be assisted Prosthetic appliance unit Visit the operating department during reconstructive surgery; Attend the outpatient's department to observe follow-up visits Attend a long-stay residential rehabilitation unit for one week's work experience Inter-personal skills: supporting people facing a long term disability through each phase of grieving; supporting the family of clients Legal and social aspects of disability: appreciate the short- and long-term implications for clients suffering injury caused by, for example: road-traffic accidents, industrial, civil damage or from war Employment issues: understand the employment law and issues regarding re-employment following injury, including workplace modifications	**Nursing learners:** Practical nursing: Prevention and recognition of potential and actual complications of immobility Promoting mobility: from bed to chair, to walk with the use of prescribed aids, to use a wheelchair safely Promoting independence through daily routines and activities such as eating and drinking, personal hygiene and dressing Treatment of medical conditions including skin lesions and prevention of infection Use of orientation strategies to promote mental health Understand the role of different members of the health and social care team **Under supervision:** develop and implement a personalised care plan for one or more clients, using the prescribed protocols; evaluate and modify care plans as needed on a daily basis; develop a discharge programme for one or more clients taking account of the full range of relevant professionals; manage the care of a small group of clients over the period of a week

These different activities reflect some of the work undertaken to support people suffering severe trauma. Some of the activities are beneficial to any learner visiting the unit, and some are profession-specific.

You will have noticed that some of the learning experiences are profession-focussed, such as developing technical and management skills, while others are more generic, and learners from any profession would benefit from a placement in the unit. In the example of Rothermead, visiting nursing learners are using generic professional skills in the specific context of the rehabilitation unit. They are also learning to recognise the relevance of book knowledge as well as their knowledge gained from earlier placements. Their generic experiences are gained by engaging with a wide range of professionals who also support the clients at Rothermead throughout their health and social care pathway. Giving learners opportunities to go on visits outside the unit provides a much deeper and more memorable learning experience than that provided by textbooks, or lectures. It helps them to understand the contribution of other members of the team. If such visits marry up with those by learners from other professions, they will all benefit from shared learning and working, thus enhancing future inter-professional understanding and communication. Table 4.5 provides you with some questions to consider and activities when developing a curriculum of practice.

Table 4.5   Developing your curriculum of practice.

---

* What profession-specific activities are available for learners to develop?
* Make a list of the different departments and organisations that link in with the work of your own workplace and that could broaden learners' understanding of your clients' health and social care pathway.
* What kind of inter-professional experiences might you include for visiting learners in your workplace?
* Are all the experiences you have identified suitable for learners at all stages of their placement?
* If you think some learners from your own profession should have different learning experiences from others, why might this be true and what are these experiences?
* Draw up a learning curriculum for your workplace for visiting learners in your own profession and try to classify the activities under different headings as in Table 4.4
* Share your curriculum with a new visiting learner and find out whether s/he has any any suggestions to make about it.

Having identified the many different kinds of learning experiences that your workplace is able to offer, you will probably find that they can be married up with the learning outcomes that visiting learners are required to achieve during their placement. Two examples are the skill clusters and Proficiencies that all nursing learners are required to achieve at different stages in their pre-registration programme. Table 4.6 illustrates this using the example given in Table 4.4.

Reading through Table 4.6 and the suggested relationship between the Rivermead Rehabilitation Learning experiences and requirements for nursing learner's professional registration (the NMC skill clusters and Proficiencies), you will see that the Proficiencies are concerned with the process in which learning is achieved rather than the detail of the experience or where it takes place. This is intended to provide flexibility within the scope of the EU Directives to programme providers and their service partners. The different placements and their learning experiences give learners the opportunity to develop and refine their knowledge and skills in a range of contexts while engaged in similar activities. The skill clusters are designed to ensure learners achieve competence in specific activities and can demonstrate their performance according to the NMC Proficiencies. It could be argued that learners do not need to change their placements as frequently as nursing programmes require, because learners could probably develop proficiency in all the prescribed areas in one or two placements. However, the requirements of the EU Directives make this impossible for nurses preparing for the adult (or general) part of the Professional register, partly because of the range of placement experiences required and partly because of the volume of learners commissioned to take the course.

Table 4.6   Application of NMC skill clusters and proficiencies.

Rothermead learning experiences	NMC skill cluster	NMC proficiency
Inter-personal skills: supporting people facing a long-term disability through each phase of grieving; supporting the family of clients; accompany residents for social outings and activities; understanding the different roles of members of the health and social care team use of planned orientation strategies to promote mental health	Care and compassion	Manage oneself, one's practice, and that of others, in accordance with The NMC code of professional conduct: standards for conduct, performance and ethics7 (the Code), recognising one's own abilities and limitations. Practise in accordance with an ethical and legal framework that ensures the primacy of patient and client interest and well-being and respects confidentiality. Practise in a fair and anti-discriminatory way, acknowledging the differences in beliefs and cultural practices of individuals or groups. Create and utilise opportunities to promote the health and well-being of patients, clients and groups.
Under close or distant supervision as assessed to be appropriate: Manage and deliver the care of a small group of clients Develop and implement a personalised care plan for one or more clients, using the prescribed protocols Evaluate and modify care plans as needed on a daily basis Develop a discharge programme for one or more clients taking account of the full range of relevant professionals	Communication	Engage in, develop and disengage from therapeutic relationships through the use of appropriate communication and interpersonal skills. Enhance the professional development and safe practice of others through peer support, leadership, supervision and teaching.
	Organisational aspects of care	Undertake and document a comprehensive, systematic and accurate nursing assessment of the physical, psychological, social and spiritual needs of patients, clients and communities Formulate and document a plan of nursing care, where possible in partnership with patients, clients, their carers and family and friends, within a framework of informed consent. Demonstrate key skills. Provide a rationale for the nursing care delivered which takes account of social, cultural, spiritual, legal, political and economic influences. Delegate duties to others, as appropriate, ensuring that they are supervised and monitored. Demonstrate knowledge of effective inter-professional working practices which respect and utilize the contributions of members of the health and social care team. Contribute to public protection by creating and maintaining a safe environment of care through the use of quality assurance and risk management strategies.

(continued)

Table 4.6   (cont'd)

Rothermead learning experiences	NMC skill cluster	NMC proficiency
		Evaluate and document the outcomes of nursing and other interventions. Demonstrate sound clinical judgement across a range of differing professional and care delivery contexts.
Professional skills: Prevent and recognise potential and actual complications of immobility Treat medical conditions including skin lesions as prescribed and prevent infection. Promote mobility: from bed to chair, to walk with the use of prescribed aids, to use a wheelchair safely. Promote independence through daily routines and activities such as eating and drinking, personal hygiene and dressing.	Infection prevention and control Nutrition and fluid maintenance Medicines management	Based on the best available evidence, apply knowledge and an appropriate repertoire of skills indicative of safe nursing practice.
Engage in the generic learning experiences identified.		Demonstrate a commitment to the need for continuing professional development and personal supervision activities in order to enhance knowledge, skills, values and attitudes needed for safe and effective nursing practice.

A common complaint by clinical staff is that they do not understand how to interpret their visiting learners' assessment schedule. If you or your colleagues have this problem, mapping the learning opportunities available in your own workplace against your profession's requirements for learner progression (you have seen an example of this in Table 4.6) will make it easier to recognise whether your learners are making progress and whether they have successfully achieved the required outcomes. Table 4.7 provides a framework for you to create a map of your own workplace.

Table 4.7   Mapping learning experiences against your own professional requirements.

Learning experiences available	Core skills required	Requirements by professional statutory organisation for qualification

Developing learning resources and making them accessible

Earlier, we emphasised the importance of the staff as a vital learning resource for visiting learners or indeed anyone who hopes to develop expertise. Many clinical staff believe that 'teaching' means a formal interactive or even didactic process where the 'holder' of the knowledge feeds the learner with information, the empty vessel approach. While this kind of exchange of information may be helpful on the rare occasion, it does not represent the knowledge that is needed in the workplace. In Chapters 5 and 6, we shall be exploring how as a practitioner you can share your professional craft/finger-tip knowledge that is so valuable. In this section, we shall look at the range of additional resources that are helpful to learners. In Table 4.4, you will have noticed several opportunities that the Rothermead rehabilitation unit made available to learners: access to the Intranet and to professional journals; opportunities to attend and participate in case conferences, to visit and potentially work in different associated departments, clinics, units and to accompany different professionals on their routines. Documenting these activities helps both staff and learners to know what is available. When you sit down with your learner to plan their placement experience, you can use your curriculum as a guide to what they can do during the first few weeks of their allocation. To create a learning plan using this information, you can include dates and times for the experiences so that both you and your learner have a record of the agreed targets. You can include a list of the different professionals who regularly work alongside the resident staff, thus offering opportunities for your learner to gain an understanding of their contribution to the care of your client group. Material resources are also a valuable means of helping your learner to become familiar with aspects of your clients' health care pathway, such as:

- case notes;
- diagnostic investigations and results;
- treatments, including medications (the drug cupboard is a fantastic resource for learning about the commonly used medications);
- time spent in the departments of related professionals, such as: therapy groups, clinics, operating department sessions, investigation departments (radiography, cardiology, etc.), outpatient departments or ante-/post-natal clinics. Sitting in on relevant clinics helps learners to understand all aspects of their client's care pathway. Attending out-patient clinics provides opportunities to see returning clients/patients as well as those presenting for the first time. After several people have been seen with similar symptoms, it becomes easier to understand their perspective of their illness (or pregnancy) and their management.
- reference books and relevant journal articles, preferably through subscription to a relevant professional journal;
- anatomical models of relevance to the clinical speciality.

Clearly, this list is not comprehensive, and it may not be particularly relevant to every kind of healthcare setting, but it provides some ideas of what you could create in your own workplace. Encouraging learners to spend time exploring these resources along with some guidance or with the help of a reference book is enormously beneficial.

Quality assurance

As with all government-funded agencies, the quality of the activities that they fund are regularly and routinely inspected and audited to ensure public monies are protected and that agencies do deliver the commissioned services and are of the required standard. Educational programmes and programme providers in the United Kingdom are audited on behalf of national Higher Education Funding Councils by a Quality Assurance Agency. Their auditors seek evidence on an annual basis that the finances and management of the institution are sound. They also conduct a six-yearly (or sometimes more frequent) visit to the institution to conduct a detailed investigation of its facilities, the quality of the learners' experiences including learning and teaching. With the focus of interest being the learner experiences, these visits always include learners' participation at informal meetings with the audit team. Learners are normally represented by colleagues from a range of programmes and who represent colleagues from different stages in their programme.

Professional programmes, such as medicine, physiotherapy, nursing and so on, are also audited by or on behalf of their relevant professional, statutory and regulatory organisation (PRSO) at regular (three-yearly) intervals to ensure that the programmes are fit for purpose and meet national and international standards. To reduce bureaucracy, these audits are often conducted by the Quality Assurance Agency for higher education and the PRSO at the same time as the subject audit. In addition, any new professional programme or remodelled programme is audited by the PRSO to assess its suitability and ability to meet their requirements before approval is given for them to be delivered.

So, for example, nursing, midwifery and health visiting programmes are seen to be a collaborative enterprise between the AEI and the service/placement providers. Quality assurance activities take place for approval of new programmes, re-approval and ongoing monitoring. These activities are conducted on behalf of the Nursing and Midwifery Council (the PRSO) by its representatives, including appropriate registrants. In an example for auditing a mental-health programme, the team would include a mental-health service manager or a practice educator, a mental-health academic and possibly a service user. These people would have received training in the audit process and be supported by a senior auditor representing the NMC. As well as inspecting the AEI, the audit team will hold several meetings with different groups, including learners, service-provider representatives including clinical managers, staff supporting learners (mentors) and, not least, patients and their carers.

Criteria that are normally used for both approval and audit events are:

- evidence of the ability of the programme to meet contemporary professional statutory requirements;
- coherence of the learners' experience;
- satisfactory provision for appropriate supervision, teaching and assessment of learners;
- provision of sufficient and appropriate placements for practice education;
- examination of practice and academic work is consistent and rigorous with appropriate external monitoring;
- internal regulation and administration of the programme is explicit, rigorous, consistent and fair.

(taken from Nursing and Midwifery Council 2010b).

Ongoing quality assurance also takes place within the education provider, which delivers an annual report to the PRSO, with evidence that these criteria are continuing to be met through its governance processes.

Part of this governance process is to monitor the effectiveness of placement providers at a local level. Each programme provider has a system for monitoring the quality of placements using a range of criteria, many of which we have already discussed in this chapter and in Chapter 3. External quality monitors will use standards for practice learning documented by the professional statutory and regulatory organisation. Table 4.8 illustrates the placement standards required for learners preparing for registration as a nurse, midwife or health visitor.

Table 4.8 Placement Learning Environment Quality Audit Criteria (NMC UK wide framework 2011).

Programme providers must ensure that:		
Supervision	**Resources**	**Assessment and documentation**
Learners are allocated to an identified mentor, practice teacher or supervisor during practice learning	Learning time is protected as specified (e.g., number of clinical hours in placement)	Information that includes dates, outcomes to be achieved and assessment documents, is made available to learners and placement supervisors
Those who supervise practice are properly prepared and supported in the role	Learning opportunities are offered at an appropriate academic level using evidence-based sources	
Those who supervise practice meet relevant requirements within the Standards to support learning and assessment in practice (SSLAinP, Nursing and Midwifery Council of the United Kingdom 2008a, b)	Learners have opportunities to learn with, and from other health and social care professionals	A variety of assessments are used to test the acquisition of approved outcomes with reasonable adjustments for learners with a disability
Local registers of mentors and practice teachers are maintained according to SSLAinP, Nursing and Midwifery Council of the United Kingdom (2008a, b)	Learners have access to a range of practice-learning opportunities sufficient to meet programme outcomes	Assessment processes enable learners to demonstrate fitness for practice and fitness for award
Objective criteria and processes are used for approving new practice-learning environments and audit them at least every 2 years.		

Nursing and Midwifery Council of the United Kingdom (2012).

Points to ponder:

Reading through Table 4.8, you might like to consider the following points:

- How does your own workplace ensure supervisors of learners are prepared and supported?
- How does your employer know who is working as a supervisor and needs continuing education?

- If you are already a supervisor, what kind of preparation did you receive for your supervisory role, and what further help would be helpful to you?
- If you are preparing to become a supervisor, what continuing support is available to you?
- To what extent are you familiar with the assessment of practice policies and strategies for the learners you support?

Being aware of the professional standards required of supervisors, and your own responsibilities towards meeting these, is as important as your employer's responsibilities towards meeting the professional standards for delivering its services and for supporting its staff in preparing the next generation of staff.

The programme provider has to be satisfied that learners are receiving high quality learning experiences both throughout the institution and throughout their practice placements. Contributing to this process are learners' evaluations of each placement experience, and evidence from placement quality-assurance monitoring activities. A vital part of learners' learning experiences is opportunities to develop professional practice to the highest standards. The service provider also has responsibility to the government to demonstrate fiscal responsibility and high standards of practice. Their clinical governance activities, to monitor service delivery and to ensure that it is of a consistently high standard, also contribute to the programme provider's monitoring information.

You will see in Table 4.8 that the standards relating to resources are focussed particularly on the kind of access learners have to practitioners' professional knowledge, and we will be exploring this in the next chapter.

Summary

In this chapter, we have explored the multitude of complex factors that influence a course curriculum leading to professional qualification. These factors originate from international, national and local policies, and are further complicated by what resources are available within participating service providers and the different placements. Your role as a supervisor or mentor is probably the most important in helping learners negotiate their way through what results from these negotiations. By developing a curriculum for your own workplace, you and your colleagues are able to communicate the important aspects of your work. This makes it easier to induct newcomers, visiting learners or new staff so as to help them feel welcomed and valued members of your community of practice. The curriculum also provides a base that you can use to advise your learners what experiences are available, as well as helping them to see how they can achieve their programme learning requirements. Establishing these kinds of structures and processes within your workplace helps you and your colleagues to meet the critical standards of the auditors representing governmental agencies and your professional organisation.

Chapter 5

Identifying your learner's needs and documenting a working learning plan

Jenny Spouse

Introduction

This chapter will focus on an exploration of your learner's needs and how these can be determined and documented. It will discuss different methods of assessing learning needs such as technical skills, knowledge and understanding, attitudes, motivation and preferred approaches to learning. We will also consider the importance of agreeing and documenting a working, learning plan and how it provides a structure for your supervisory activities. An increasingly important influence on your learner's success is early diagnosis of factors that might affect their learning needs such as people with dyslexia, sight loss or mental-health needs. Without effective support, all learners can fail to make the kind of progress of which they are capable. So, we will suggest a range of practice-related activities that you can use to help your learners to maximise their abilities and to be successful. Contributing theoretical grounding to the chapter will be an analysis and discussion of some snapshots and vignettes of practice supervision where we draw on some theories of how people learn.

This chapter includes the following:

- sponsorship to the community of practice;
- exploring and explaining socialisation;
- identifying and assessing learning needs – the components and some strategies;
- writing a working learning plan, its uses and abuses;
- exploring and explaining theories of how people learn; self-determination theory;
- meeting the needs of learners with disabilities: promoting inclusivity, diversity and equality;
- supporting learners with dyslexia, sensory impairment or mental-health needs.

Sponsorship to a community of practice

In Chapters 3 and 4, we explored the different factors that can influence the quality of a workplace as an effective learning environment. In this chapter, we look at how you can capitalise on the resources within your workplace to the benefit of learners, either new

Practice-Based Learning in Nursing, Health and Social Care: Mentorship, Facilitation and Supervision,
First Edition. Ian Scott and Jenny Spouse.
© 2013 John Wiley & Sons, Ltd. Published 2013 by John Wiley & Sons, Ltd.

staff or visiting learners. Both groups of learners will be keen to feel part of the social network and to make a contribution to the work of your team. It is their only route to feeling accepted and valued. Helping them to achieve this social acceptance in a community of practice is their participation in everyday activities. However, their participation needs to be both meaningful and thus appropriate to their capabilities and learning needs. For these learners, the most important member of the community of practice is the person who acts as their sponsor. Normally, a sponsor should be a senior member of the community who is able to orientate the newcomers to the workplace and who can ensure they receive the support that they need, either through their own efforts or by delegating supervisory responsibility to a different team member. If newcomers fail to receive sponsorship, they are likely to leave the organisation within six months. Visiting learners who are allocated to a placement have little choice over whether they stay or leave, unless they also quit their programme and thus jeopardise their career aspirations. A further complication for visiting learners is their placement-assessment documentation of their progress. Most learners wanting to become professionally qualified will need it to have a good end-of-placement report. Vignette 5.1 provides an illustration of sponsorship.

Vignette 5.1   Gareth's experiences of sponsorship

Gareth is starting his second clinical placement on a surgical ward in a large teaching hospital. The practice educator for the surgical unit has given him joining instructions, including the name of his mentor and that he is to attend for the 1'o clock afternoon shift.

Arriving a little earlier, he finds the ward manager and introduces himself. She shows him where to store his belongings, as there are no communal staff lockers, and introduces him to the person who will be his mentor (Lucy). Lucy is a senior staff nurse and has worked on the ward for the past five years. She has recently completed a Master's degree in advanced practice; she also holds a teaching certificate from her local further education college. In the short time before shift handover, Lucy takes him around the ward, introduces him to the staff on duty and shows him the layout. She shows him where the policies and protocols are stored and how to use the computer system. Patient notes and charts are all online. They then go to sit in on the shift handover. As Lucy will be the senior nurse for the shift, she introduces Gareth to a colleague, Mitch, who will be co-mentoring him during his placement and specifically that afternoon. At the end of handover, Mitch chats to Gareth finding out what he hopes to achieve during the placement and how he got on in his first placement. Gareth has remembered to bring his placement passport for Mitch to see what he actually achieved as well as the learning outcomes he needs to achieve during this placement. This takes about half an hour, and as most of the patients are having an afternoon rest, they can afford the time.

When they have finished chatting, Mitch takes Gareth on his nursing round, chatting to their group of patients to assess their needs, whether they need further analgesia and how they feel about their recovery from surgery, and checking their wound and paper charts. A few of the patients have returned from surgery in the morning.

During their round, Mitch has been observing Gareth's behaviour, whether he is relaxed and respectful towards the patients, how much he appears to understand about the surgical procedures and the medications patients are receiving, his overall level of confidence and so on. For the rest of the afternoon, the two of them work together with Gareth participating fully in the different activities by supporting Mitch. After suppers have been served and during visiting time, the two of them sit down and discuss Gareth's observations of the patients and his feelings about the shift. Mitch asks Gareth to go away with a copy of the ward's learning curriculum of experiences and to return the next day with his placement plan, that is, the things he wants to learn and the experiences he wants to have.

Points to ponder:

- How do you think Gareth felt about his first shift on the ward?
- What do you think about the arrangements that Lucy made for Gareth?
- Thinking about the shift that Mitch and Gareth spent together, what do you think Mitch might report to Lucy about Gareth?
- If you were Mitch, what might you plan to do with Gareth on his next shift?

Vignette 5.1 illustrates a number of important processes that facilitate entry to a community of practice, which we will explore through the eyes of the visiting learner, Gareth.

Gareth most probably felt thrilled and relieved that the placement staff were actually expecting him and had taken the trouble to make preparations for him. As a result, he has been able to meet his mentor as well as his appointed co-mentor (Mitch). Being able to work closely with him is a great advantage, as his main mentor, Lucy, is likely to be pre-occupied with managing the ward. Although Gareth may not remember where everything is stored on the ward, by being shown around he has been given tacit permission to find the whereabouts of things for himself. In the same manner, everyone on the shift has now met him, and because his mentor is a respected senior member of staff, they will look after him. This provides Gareth with sponsorship, and as a result Gareth will have positive feelings about working and learning on the placement. This kind of sponsorship has also given Gareth an identity within this new community of practitioners and allowed him to feel valued. An experience like this is highly motivating, and it is likely that Gareth will be enthusiastic about studying as much as possible about the clinical speciality: surely a win–win outcome. Several researchers, who were sociologists, have investigated how learners develop their professional knowledge. They described the learning process as socialisation to the workplace environment.

Exploring and explaining socialisation and learning to become a professional

Theories from different theoretical disciplines explaining how people learn in society, such as sociology (Mead 1934; Habermas 1984), educational psychology (Dewey 1939; Piaget 1972) and socio-cultural theories (Vygotsky 1978; Wertsch 1991) suggest that it is best achieved through contact with members of their community.

Learning how to conform to the normal behaviour of an important social group is defined as socialisation. In the United States, the Chicago school of sociologists significantly influenced our understanding of adult and professional socialisation; in particular, the influence of the Chicago sociologist, Herbert Mead, and his belief that through seeing the self as an object, humans come to measure their ideal image and actual performance against others (Mead 1934). Another important contribution to current understanding of adult socialisation has been the work of Brim and Wheeler (1966). Brim argues that role acquisition is the most important aspect of adult socialisation and correlates it with personality change, a profound and perhaps most painful adjustment made in life (Brim 1966: 6). Learning how to adjust personal actions so that they match those of the 'important' people around you is more likely to be successful by engaging with those people and internalising the process.

Most people can distinguish a stranger or a tourist from a local person. A stranger tends to be instantly noticeable, often by the way they dress, their behaviour and nuances of their vocabulary or accent. The same can be said about groups of young people, who tend to dress in the same fashions and use the same kinds of language. In common with them are different professional groups and sub-groups who may be distinguished by shared and often unique characteristics such as customary practices, mode of dress, use of language, their vocabulary, the short-hand terms and abbreviations used to describe common events or situations, all of which are hallmarks of shared values. These characteristics ensure every member of the community knows what behaviour is acceptable, thus promoting order and stability to the community (Brim and Wheeler 1966; Schutz 1970; Bourdieu 1991). Unconsciously, these unique characteristics of a community will bond its members together, making it difficult for newcomers to become part of the community until they adopt and understand the specialist characteristics of the community. Socialisation is thus more than the outward adaptation of cultural trappings but the ability to take on the beliefs, attitudes and language of the community into your own personal practice.

For visiting learners to survive each of their health or social practice placements, they have to adjust to each different community of practice that they visit. They have to learn the language of the setting as well as the practices and modes of being of that setting, while retaining their academic knowledge and values. Often, newcomers or visiting learners have to reconcile their personal images of how they see themselves in their professional role with the images presented by their academic learning and their experiences in their practice placements. In their desire to be successful, learners have to adapt to the official perspective and employ strategies to take on the values of those with whom they wish to be successful. It is not unusual for learners to find there are significant differences in belief systems between the academic and their placements colleagues (Davis 1975). Much later, a Canadian study of undergraduate nursing learners by Day and colleagues (Day et al. 1995) found that their learners experienced the same kinds of differences. As learners spent more time in 'the real world' of practice, so they came to espouse the attitudes and behaviours of their clinical colleagues. American sociologist Ida Harper Simpson's pioneering ethnographic study of nurse socialisation, undertaken in the late 1950s, investigated learners taking a four-year university degree programme. Using Piaget's (1896–1980) human development model, she identified socialisation as a three-stage transitional process, moving from technical skill orientation, through interpersonal orientation to key members of the practice arena to internalisation of professional values (Simpson 1967).

In her sociological study of Scottish learner nurses, Kath Melia (1987) noticed very similar processes experienced by her participants. She identified five major stages in her learners' socialisation, calling the stages: fitting in; learning the rules; getting the work done; learning and working; and passing through. Melia described how learners believed their survival depended upon their ability to conform to the culture of each placement (Melia 1987). A summary of the main findings from these three studies is illustrated in Table 5.1. You may find yourself considering your own experiences of being a learner and whether these models have relevance to them.

Melia's (1987) themes reflect the itinerant nature of learners and their felt necessity to fit into each clinical community, while trying to extract sufficient knowledge and skills to be worthy of qualification. Melia also found that learners spent considerable time in each new placement trying to identify their ward sister's preferences as well as those of the rest of the staff (Melia 1987). Because learners rely heavily upon the support of the clinical staff to engage them in their everyday practice and thus their progress, they felt they had to hide any feelings of disagreement or dissonance with what they observed or were asked

Table 5.1 Comparison of three models of how nurses learn to be a nurse.

Researcher study time and publication epistemology	Ida Harper Simpson study in 1950s published 1967 ethnography/SI	Fred Davis study 1962–1964 published 1968 ethnography/SI	Kath Melia PhD study 1981 published 1987 ethnography/SI
Stages of socialisation	Transition from lay to technical/procedural	Initial innocence	Fitting in
	Task orientation	Labelled recognition of incongruity	Learning the rules
	Attachment to significant others	Psyching out	Getting the work done
		Role simulation	Learning and working
	Internalisation of professional values	Provisional internalisation	Just passing through
		Stable internalisation	

to do (Luker 1984). A number of UK studies investigating nursing learner' wastage found the most consistent reason for leaving their programme was the difficulties they experienced when struggling to cope in practice placements, with these kinds of socialisation processes (MacGuire 1970; Wyatt 1978; Parkes 1985).

It is not unusual for learners to be faced with a moral conflict, especially when their academic study has taught them to deliver care on the basis of research evidence, and they find that such research has not permeated the clinical scene. Mackay (1989), and later May et al. (1997), a decade later, researching nurse education in England illustrated how learners often adopted outdated attitudes and practices from their clinical supervisors in order to survive (Mackay 1989; May et al. 1997). Similar findings have been found in studies of how medical learners and foundation year doctors cope when entering their clinical placements (Chittenden et al. 2009). High levels of stress are an unnecessary and avoidable price learners have to pay in order to survive within an environment that is unfavourable or unwelcoming towards incoming learners.

Researching nursing education in the United Kingdom in the 1980s, Bradby observed that many learners became confused when they were called 'nurse' before they felt able to identify with that title (Bradby 1990: 1223). This is largely concerned with the extent to which learners are able to function in the same manner as their 'professional' colleagues within the community of practice. If they were undertaking the same kinds of activities as their nursing colleagues, they were more likely to feel part of the team and to feel that they were doing nursing work (Spouse 2003a, b). These sociological interpretations of how people normally behave in order to survive an unfamiliar environment provide some explanations of how visiting learners cope with frequent changes of placement.

Reading through Vignette 5.1, it seems as though Gareth is lucky; he has a mentor who is a respected member of the community of practice and who has delegated some of her mentorship responsibilities to a colleague who seems well prepared to look after a new member of their community. Mitch has taken time to engage with Gareth and to get to know him and his approach to caring for patients. From a sociological perspective, Gareth is in a good position to benefit from the placement, because he has been sponsored into the community of practice by a senior member of staff. He has been given status by his mentor and co-mentor and so other staff members will recognise him as needing, perhaps worthy, of their support. Gareth also has at least two named people to whom he can go for help, to work alongside and thus learn from. In the ideal situation, Gareth will see staff using evidence to support their clinical actions and thus find congruence between his academic and clinical learning.

Identifying and assessing learning needs – the components and some strategies

To help Gareth achieve the most from his placement, Mitch needs to find out what Gareth is capable of doing safely and what he needs to learn during his placement. There are two important reasons why assessing Gareth's level of capability is essential.

First, Mitch has a duty of care towards the patients under his care along with Lucy, Gareth's mentor and the ward sister. They have a duty of care towards anyone who comes into the ward. Thus, they would put these people (including Gareth) at risk if they delegated duties to Gareth without knowing whether he was competent to undertake them.

Second, Gareth has come to the placement with specific goals. Unless he is able to undertake duties that help him to achieve these goals, he will either fail this specific placement or fail subsequent placements because he has not developed the necessary foundation knowledge and skills.

During Gareth's first shift when he worked alongside Mitch, he was able to demonstrate his professional and personal skills, such as motivation and willingness to learn, level of self-consciousness and self awareness, confidence, ability to relate to the patients and ability to undertake delegated tasks effectively. How was Mitch able to detect these attributes from Gareth? Table 5.2 illustrates some assumptions that Mitch could reasonably have made.

Table 5.2   Assessing professional and personal attributes.

Professional skills	Gareth arrived on duty before the start of shift, dressed correctly and looking tidy and smart, clean shoes and uniform. He had clearly prepared himself for the placement, as he knew the names of senior staff and the clinical specialities of the ward. His manner was polite and respectful to everyone that he met, and he spoke sensitively to patients and their relatives.

Personal skills:
  Motivation
  Willingness to learn
	His preparation for the placement came through in the kinds of questions that he asked, and the level of knowledge that he displayed.
	He took notice of what he was told and asked thoughtful questions at appropriate times.

Level of self-consciousness	During the handover, it was clear that Gareth was a bit awed by the process and tended to keep in the background. His body language at times suggested he was not yet (quite naturally) comfortable in his new surroundings.
Level of self-awareness	When describing his previous placement, Gareth was open and honest, and acknowledged that he had been struggling to adjust to his new career and the discipline of working and studying.
Ability to take on delegated tasks	When Mitch asked him to fetch items, or to assist in some of the care delivery, Gareth undertook the tasks, with grace and willingness, and completed them promptly.

On his second shift, Mitch needs to take a deeper look at Gareth's abilities, and together they need to develop a learning plan or agenda for his placement, or at least the first half of Gareth's placement. Vignette 5.2 illustrates how Mitch went about the assessment part of this process.

Vignette 5.2   Working together for assessment

Gareth returned to the ward next day, confident in knowing that he would be working alongside Mitch for the morning shift. After the preliminary handover, together they went around all their team of patients to see how they were and to assess their nursing needs and plan their own work.

Some people were fasting prior to surgery, while others needed immediate treatment, and others were mostly self-caring or wanted to rest a bit longer. This information helped Mitch to plan and to prioritise his work for the morning. Normally, Mitch would have made his plans mentally, but as he was teaching Gareth how to manage his workload, Mitch took the trouble to make his plans overt. First, he made a list of the activities they needed to do for each patient, along with an estimated time it would take. As a result of their nursing round, they were able to identify their priorities and to agree with each patient an approximate time they would go to them. Their nursing plan included an account for the different visiting professionals who would be attending the patients, and the preparation any patients needed if going for investigations or for surgery later in the day. By Mitch making his thinking explicit, he was providing a framework for Gareth to see how he could plan his own work. They then agreed how Gareth would assist Mitch in these activities.

Their first actions were to administer analgesics to all the people who needed them. Some patients received a small dose intravenously so that it would work quickly, while others had intramuscular or oral analgesia. In this process, Gareth was able to learn how to check prescriptions, to learn something about analgesia, and to learn how to draw up and administer intramuscular injections. While the analgesia was taking effect, they checked those patients preparing for surgery to make sure everything was in order. Then, together, they went back to the most ill patients to make a thorough assessment of their condition (wound, drainage tubes, vital signs, etc.) and to give them their morning wash, change their bed and help them to sit out of bed while it was made fresh. During this process, Gareth provided assistance to Mitch. The second patient they went to, the roles reversed, and Gareth took the lead with Mitch assisting him. Over the morning shift, the pair worked in this manner, Mitch demonstrating while Gareth assisted, followed by Gareth taking the lead with Mitch coaching him. During their 11 am coffee break together, they discussed what they had been doing. This gave Gareth an opportunity to ask questions.

At the end of the shift, prior to formally documenting their activities, Mitch asked Gareth to write up a draft report of their morning activities to go into the patients' notes. They then spent time discussing what he had written and agreed on what would go into the notes.

Points to ponder:

- What do you think about this approach to assessing and teaching?
- What do you think Mitch learned about Gareth during this shift?
- What kinds of things might Mitch discuss with Gareth when they come to make a learning plan?
- What do you think of the way Mitch worked with Gareth?

Over the shift described in Vignette 5.2, Mitch was able to observe how Gareth related to the patients, how quickly he was able to learn unfamiliar information and skills, and how much of his academic learning he was able to bring to his practice. He could see whether Gareth knew how to use a wide range of technical skills while caring for their patients and, during their conversations together, was able to make a note of aspects that he needed to develop further. Perhaps the most important thing that Mitch was determining was the extent to which Gareth knew his own limitations, whether he understood the implications of what he was doing and whether he could be trusted to report back to him if he had any concerns.

From Gareth's perspective, he was doing what he hoped he would be doing during this placement, which was to learn from an experienced practitioner, to have access to his professional knowledge, the tips and tactics, and to be able to develop the necessary skills and knowledge to make a reciprocal contribution to the team as a 'thank you' for the time they were investing in him.

From a sociological perspective, Gareth was being made to feel a part of the team (fitting in), he had sponsorship into the community of practice (attachment to significant others), he was being legitimately involved in everyday activities that were important to the delivery of care of the patients, and so he felt that he was being valued as an individual and his needs as a learner were being respected.

Writing a working learning plan, its uses and abuses

After lunch, Mitch and Gareth returned to the ward and spent some time discussing a learning plan for the first half of his placement. The previous evening, Gareth had taken a copy of the Ward Opportunities for Learning, a catalogue of activities and places he could visit during his placement. Mitch and Gareth would use this for their planning. At the end of an hour, they had drawn up a plan that looked like that shown in Table 5.3.

Reading through this plan, it looks very straightforward, possibly common sense and, some might even say, unnecessary. However, having a plan of action documented like this one for Gareth formalises and identifies that he is a learner with needs. It legitimises his need for support, in the form of close supervision, continuous assessment and coaching from his mentors and their colleagues. It also illustrates what a lot he has to achieve in four weeks. The level at which he will be expected to function is defined by the level of dependency of the patients he will care for while under more distant supervision.

Being afforded opportunities to leave the ward, first to accompany a patient to theatre and to observe their operation and post-operative recovery, helps Gareth understand what has happened to the patient and why they need analgesia as well as the kinds of post-operative complication they could experience. The experience also helps him to learn how to care for patients through this critical stage in their illness. A second visit allows him to see a range of operations and to begin to appreciate how an operating department functions. The visit to the outpatient department provides a range of educational experiences linked to the clinical speciality, thus enriching his understanding of the speciality and, more importantly, the health care pathway patients have and will experience.

Overall, having a learning plan demonstrates three important aspects:

- It is a commitment from the clinical team to support Gareth in his learning and prescribes the level of achievement that they believe is reasonable to expect of him at his stage in his programme, his assessed level of capability and the time available.

Table 5.3   Gareth's learning plan for the first 4 weeks of his placement.

Skills and knowledge: be able to	Activities
Prepare a patient for surgery, that is, describe the information required by the patient about the surgery, including assessment, fasting and hygiene preparation	Work alongside Mitch with a range of patients until competent to deliver care to patients with 'low to medium' dependency under more distant supervision
Accompany a patient to surgery and to remain with them throughout, until return to the ward	Accompany a patient with Mitch to OD and stay with the patient throughout the surgery to recovery room, as an observer – to be arranged for week 2 of placement
Deliver post-operative care to patients including: observation of vital signs; management of pain, management of wound and drains, etc., know how to advise the patients about prevention of post-operative complications; assisting with mobilisation effectively	Work alongside Mitch with a range of patients, until competent to deliver post-operative care to patients of 'low to medium' dependency under more distant supervision
Demonstrate understanding of, and be able to prepare patients for, specific investigations	Work alongside Mitch, until competent to prepare patients according to their care plan under more distant supervision
Become familiar with and administer commonly used drugs given by: Intramuscular injection Oral administration	Participate in drug administration: give intramuscular drugs and oral drugs under supervision at all opportunities and document accurately; during quiet times, learn about the drugs in common usage by going through the drug cupboard with BNF and pharmacopoeia; keep a drug notebook
Take and record vital signs accurately and to understand the implications of readings outside the normal range; become competent in taking blood pressure, pulse and respirations	Take and record the vital signs of all patients in team 4-hourly or as required – ongoing
Visit the operating dept.	Spend a shift observing in the operating department when patients from the ward go for surgery – to be arranged with theatre manager – in week 3
Visit to the OPD	Spend a shift in surgeons' outpatient clinic in week 4
Document nursing actions of patients accurately and promptly	With the support of Mitch, write a draft nursing report of each patient whom he has nursed at the end of each shift

- It gives him a clear agenda for his placement experience and thus a legitimate claim on the professional knowledge of the clinical team.
- It provides a measure against which Gareth's achievements can be assessed at the end of the agreed period. If, for any reason, Gareth's progress is less than hoped for, this can be documented, and the next stage of the plan will be to document the kind of remedial help he will receive. If all goes well, and Gareth demonstrates he is capable in these areas, then a more complex plan will be developed.

Exploring and explaining theories of how people learn

Throughout the process of assessment and planning Gareth's learning, Mitch was either consciously or pre-consciously drawing on a range of theories about how people learn. Probably, none of these theories provide a unique and all-encompassing explanation, but all of them can contribute to our understanding. The range of theories includes the educational psychology of humanists such as Carl Rogers, the socio-cultural theories of Lev Vygotsky, Jean Lave and Etienne Wenger, and the behaviourist theories of Skinner and Gagné. Using learning theories to analyse assumptions implicit in Vignette 5.2 and Table 5.3, we can see how the humanistic learning theories of Carl Rogers help to explain the work that Mitch and Gareth have carried out during Gareth's first 24 h on the ward.

Table 5.4   Using learning theories to analyse assumptions implicit in Vignette 5.2 and Table 5.3.

Actions	Analysis
Gareth was invited to take the Menu of Learning Opportunities (LO) home and to return with a wish list for the first 4 weeks of his placement; from this wish list, he and his mentor, Mitch, planned Gareth's first 4 weeks of placement	Gareth knew the criteria for his placement, and these provided boundaries of any choices that he could make, that is, achievement of his placement learning outcomes in the context of surgical nursing. However, the Menu of LO for the placement indicated there was scope for Gareth to make decisions about what aspects of surgical nursing he would particularly like to learn about during his placement. He was encouraged by his mentor to negotiate when he could reasonably have the experiences, thus giving a measure of autonomy. Carl Rogers, an educational psychologist, identifies factors that influence whether adults learn, and these include the ability to be self-determining by making choices relevant to personal need. Along with other theorists, he argues that humans need to see the object of their learning as a means towards achieving personal goals.

Exploring and explaining Humanistic theories of how adults learn

Carl Rogers (1902–1987) was a psychotherapist who, from his own experiences and research, developed a theory that made his client the centre of the therapeutic transaction. Carl Rogers later applied his theory to education, describing it as learner-centred (see Rogers 1983). Rogers argued that people learn best when they are committed to the subject and have control over the content and pace of their learning. This humanistic approach to how people can be helped to learn transformed approaches to education in the West and has led to an understanding that learning is a life-long process rather than a process of 'filling an empty vessel' with knowledge. In the past, teachers had seen themselves as having sole responsibility for determining what was learned and when it should take place, hence the metaphor of people as empty vessels waiting to be filled by their teachers with knowledge. Following the work of Rogers, as well as other educational theorists, educationalists came to see teachers as facilitators of learning and the learner as having the responsibility for their own learning. Teachers, in every context, continue to have an important role in supporting learning. In practice placement settings, this includes identifying and designing a programme of learning (a curriculum) that meets specific needs. The Menu of Learning Opportunities available on Gareth's placement is one kind of curriculum, as it offers experiences that will engage learners in educational activities relevant to their placement and that can lead to their professional development.

Rogers (1983) argued that when people had developed an interest in a subject – such as their career aspirations, they were more likely to take responsibility for their own learning. Thus, they had an incentive to learn, and their learning was more enduring, as they perceived it to be relevant to their own needs. Complementing Rogers' approach is self-determination theory. This argues that motivation to become 'self actualised' (Maslow 1954) or to become a psychologically and emotionally integrated person influences human behaviour and the wish to learn. This intrinsic motivation, such as the desire to become a successful learner and to learn as much about the placement speciality as possible will motivate Gareth to learn and is characterised by three specific human needs: autonomy, competence and psychological relatedness (Ryan & Deci 2000). Like Carl Rogers, they believe that human beings have an innate desire to learn and to grow emotionally and intellectually while being actively and emotionally involved with other people. To achieve this, humans need to be able to pursue areas of their life that they find interesting. But this can only be achieved in a social environment that is supportive and constructive. Deci and Ryan (1985) found that extrinsic motivation often had only a short-lasting influence on motivation to learn or to conform to required behaviours. The length of time external motivation was influential depended upon the extent to which individuals have any control over their actions or are committed to the external rules and regulations. An example of rules that are frequently flouted is related to the wearing of uniform. The rules are intended to produce a standard of appearance that suggests discipline and quality. They are also designed to protect both the public and the uniform wearer from harm. However, these rules are often ignored either because wearers resent the perceived infringement on their right to self-expression or from ignorance of the purpose of the rules. When people understand the value of uniform rules and how they relate to their own personal goals, they are more likely to respect them. The same is true of promoting internal motivation when an important learning experience appears to be unrelated and boring. If learners fail to recognise the importance of a topic, such as interpersonal skills (believing they know all there is about the matter), having the topic presented in meaningful way by which learners are fully engaged increases internal motivation and thus their motivation to participate and to learn (Jang 2008).

Exploring and explaining self-determination theory applied to Gareth's experience

Gareth had considerable autonomy in this situation, in that he chose to become a registered nurse as a means of achieving his ambition to make a meaningful contribution to society, and to have job that was socially respected. He chose the particular university to take his preparatory programme, knowing where his placements were likely to take place. The external motivating factors (i.e. those imposed by the professional statutory organisation and the university) were the requirement by his programme to successfully achieve various pre-determined learning outcomes for the placement. Specific motivators for the placement are requirements that Gareth develops competence in a range of surgical nursing activities and to achieve a satisfactory report of his progress from his mentors. As these requirements are essential to Gareth's success as a registered nurse and so congruent with his own needs and ambitions, he is motivated to accept them.

Prior to his allocation, Gareth knew a little about the clinical speciality, so he had some concept about his placement. The most likely important intrinsic motivating factors are his need to achieve his learning outcomes and to be socially accepted by the community of practice. By giving Gareth a framework (the placement learning curriculum) with which to make decisions about his learning during the first four weeks of the placement, Mitch was communicating several important motivational messages:

- You are welcome to this community of practice (part of a social group).
- We are interested in you as a person, and we want to help you to succeed (being valued).
- We recognise that you will learn better if we encourage you to take responsibility for your own learning (given a reasonable level of autonomy).
- We are giving you a choice and offering you support to learn about some aspects of our clinical speciality at a different pace from others (given a reasonable level of autonomy).

Gareth's plan of work for the first four weeks includes several 'routine' and inevitably repetitive activities, such as preparing patients for surgery, accompanying patients to the operating department, conducting and recording post-operative assessments of their recovery, and providing essential post-operative care. However, Gareth can see that by conducting these routine procedures on a wide range of patients undergoing different types of surgery, he will be become very familiar with the routine of such procedures, and so he will be able to develop his competence. He will also be able to learn about the nuances of basic care plans, such as why an 18-year-old has different pre- and post-operative needs than those of an 80-year-old undergoing the same surgery.

Having time out from the general routine of the ward to visit the related departments gives Gareth a different perspective of the clinical speciality, broadening his understanding of the experiences his patients are likely to have had both prior to admission and after discharge from hospital. Such experiences also convey to Gareth that the staff recognise he is there as a learner and that his learning takes place not only through routine and regular work activities but also through these visits. Overall, the clinical team have planned for learners and are able to address their individual learning needs, which makes the placement an exemplary learning environment.

Meeting the needs of learners with special needs: promoting diversity, inclusivity and equality

Let us consider a slightly different situation where you have a learner who does not seem able to function as well as you expect (Vignette 5.3).

Vignette 5.3   Julie, a second-year learner

Julie is on a specialist placement for four weeks. Her Practice Portfolio indicates that she has been struggling to make progress, with drug administration being particularly highlighted. Julie acknowledges that her marks for academic work are very disappointing, as she has been studying hard. This is evident from her knowledge of the speciality and the quality of her relationships with her patients. During the first week of her placement, her mentor, Michael, has noticed that she is bright and asks pertinent questions; she also seems to grasp principles quickly, although sometimes seems stuck for words. In her clinical work, Julie often seems to spend an unusually long time organising her case load, not managing her time as well as would be normally expected or setting priorities effectively. When asked to go to a different department in the Unit, Julie took much longer than expected, and she explained she had got lost. Several of her colleagues were sceptical about this explanation, but it had been supported by a comment from a senior manager who had found her wandering along a corridor a long way from her destination.

Michael's suspicions that Julie has a specific problem were further aroused when he and Julie worked together to give out medications. He notices that she reads prescriptions using a small pocket ruler as a guide on each page and that it takes her longer than expected to decide what has been prescribed. When he asks her about this, Julie explains that she has difficulty reading text, as it often appears to have stripes running down it (where the spaces between the letters form patterns); the letters appear to move, and she sometimes has difficulty distinguishing between some letters. She finds reading particularly difficult when she is in a noisy environment or when there are many distractions.

Michael has dyslexia and was diagnosed when he first started his training at university; he wonders whether this might be Julie's problem and discusses his thoughts with her, sharing his own experiences.

Disability in the workplace

It is estimated that approximately 18% of the working population, or 10 million people, have a disability of some form (Health & Safety Executive 2012). UK Government legislation is designed to help as many disabled people get into work and to enjoy useful and productive lives. All employers in the United Kingdom are required by the Disability and Equality Act (HM Government 2010) to make reasonable adjustments for employees who have a disability such as dyslexia while ensuring that they come to no harm as a result of their disability. This legislation requires both the disabled person and the employer to take all reasonable steps to ensure their safety. The discussion about what is reasonable is difficult to define but often results in making the workplace a safer place for all the workers. Employers have a wide range of government organisations, such as the Health and Safety Executive and Job Centre Plus, to provide advice and support when employing disabled people. In addition, larger organisations normally have an occupational health department with a Disability Employment Advisor who provides guidance on suitable adjustments to make it possible for new staff or for learners to work safely. The NHS is considered to be a leader in employing people with a disability because of its expertise in supporting such people as well as offering role models to patients with similar problems because of their special knowledge and experience. More often than not, by making adjustments for people with disability, the rest of the community also benefit. A good example is the very small font size on many labels and posters, which defeat a large percentage of population; another is the provision of ramps to give access to wheelchair users or people using crutches.

If your workplace is going to receive a visiting learner or a new member of staff who has a disability, it is often helpful to contact your occupational therapy department and possibly the physiotherapy department for advice on any adjustments and supportive strategies that need to be made. It is very likely that a visiting learner with a disability will already possess a range of equipment to help them work and learn in a health care setting. In Vignette 5.3, Julie was unaware of the true nature of her difficulties and so needed a diagnosis so that she could access professional help.

Supporting learners with dyslexia

In the United Kingdom, approximately 6% of all schoolchildren have dyslexia, and probably at least 4% of the general population have a significant disability, while approximately 6% have a milder form. Many people miss being diagnosed as dyslexic while they are at school (British Dyslexia Association 2012, NHS 2012), and so in a society that values written abilities, they often suffer from poor self-regard. The disorder, if it can be called that, is a 'diversity of the neurological system' that affects the development of literacy and language-related skills. Its affects are likely to have been present since birth and will affect the person throughout their life. People who are affected by dyslexia will have had difficulty recognising the sounds of words and their use in different situations. Julie (in Vignette 5.3) has described some of the characteristic symptoms that people experience. People who have dyslexia are often very talented and have other skills that can be exceptional, such as millionaire and business entrepreneur, Richard Branson; Steve Jobs, founder of Apple computers and the iPhone; musicians such as John Lennon and Nigel Kennedy; scientists such as Albert Einstein and Michael Faraday; writers, artists and designers such as Agatha Christie, Roald Dahl, Leonardo da Vinci, Tommy Hilfiger, Olympic gold medallist, Sir Steven Redgrave, and television chef and entrepreneur, Jamie Oliver. These successful and famous people were able to develop strategies that either masked their dyslexia or helped them to manage the symptoms successfully. Learners who are having difficulty with their literacy and language skills often try to deny they have a problem and as a result suffer needlessly. The kinds of characteristics learners with dyslexia may demonstrate are listed in Box 5.1. You may recognise some of the characteristics as typical of your own experiences, as well as those of your learners or your colleagues, so the list is not exclusive to people with dyslexia.

In the situation encountered by Michael and Julie, they agree that she should be assessed for dyslexia by contacting the learner services centre and her professional tutor at the university, where they can arrange a psychological assessment. The tests will show whether Julie has dyslexia and the extent of her disability. She can be offered some guidance on how to use a range of tools that will help her with her studies. In the meantime, Michael and Julie try out some simple strategies that she may find helpful:

- using a coloured transparent sheet to cover written information – she needs to find out a colour that works best for her;

Box 5.1   Characteristics of learners with dyslexia.

Shows signs of tiredness
Fragile self-esteem
May show signs of stress, frustration or anger
May find reading and writing tasks tiring
Difficulty in remembering what has been read and may need to re-read for full
   understanding
Misinterpreting questions
Left/right confusion
Has difficulty with instructions about organising or processing
Has problems with managing time
Has a short concentration span/easily distracted
Difficulty with expressing ideas and concepts both verbally and in writing
May jumble up or reverse the order of numbers or letters when writing, for example, door
   codes, telephone numbers
Prefers to learn from experience or through visual strategies for example, spidergrams,
   diagrams, etc.
Has problems carrying out several tasks at once, for example, listening and writing notes
Can think creatively and use lateral thinking for problem-solving
Has good practical skills
Is resourceful and ingenious in using self
Has good analytical and problem-solving skills
Is good at public speaking and interpersonal relationships
Is proficient in making intuitive links and coming up with imaginative ideas

---

Source: Hutchinson & Atkinson (2010). With kind permission from The Chartered Society of Physiotherapists.

- using a reading pen for unfamiliar words;
- having verbal as well as written instructions, and to read out aloud when going through documents;
- developing skill in using diagrams, mind-maps, flow charts and pictograms to summarise information and to document instructions such as work plans and to create prompt sheets;
- using a digital recorder;
- using mnemonic devices and acronyms to remember names and numbers;
- using a calculator;
- carrying a pocket notebook or her mobile phone memory pad to record unfamiliar names of procedures, drugs and personnel (ensuring confidentiality is maintained);
- carrying a small alphabetical indexed book to record the names of drugs, procedures and unfamiliar words;
- becoming familiar with the different forms used in the setting, by studying them quietly alone.

Michael agreed to help her by:

- giving her instructions one at a time and, where possible, in a quiet location;
- simplifying instructions by using simple sentences and language;
- writing down important information using diagrams or flow charts;
- supporting her while she takes notes or uses a digital recorder;

- encouraging her to check her understanding by repeating instructions;
- building work planning time into her workload;
- helping her to plan her work so that she can achieve each task according to priority;
- demonstrating clinical activities more than once and getting Julie to talk through the activity until she is able to practise them independently;
- encouraging Julie to write a draft of any reports she needs to make and, where possible, provide a template or guidelines so she knows what is required.

In the United Kingdom, you can find further guidelines and information from special web sites linked to the Nursing and Midwifery Council of the United Kingdom (http://www.nmc-uk.org) or the Chartered Society of Physiotherapists (http://www.csp.org.uk/), which has an excellent handbook covering a wide range of disabilities.

Reading through these two lists of adjustments that Michael and Julie made, you can appreciate that in order to be successful, the 'reasonable adjustments' did not demand a great deal of time or effort from the clinical staff. Most of the adjustments are minor, and Julie can manage them independently but with the full support of her mentor, Michael. The most important adjustment is the attitudes of the staff working and supporting learners with special needs. You may be able to recognise that many of the actions would be just as useful to other learners, and so it would be good to adopt such practices as a matter of improving the quality of mentoring.

In Julie's situation, her dyslexia was manageable by seeking an accurate diagnosis and accepting the support offered, by using various strategies and tools available. Sometimes, learners with dyslexia go unnoticed and manage very well. Other learners have so much difficulty with interpreting important documents, such as drug prescriptions, that they are a danger to their patients and so cannot be judged as 'fit to practise' and thus cannot proceed to professional registration in their career. Tragic and difficult decisions such as this are only taken after the learner has received documented support that has not resulted in the progress needed for success, and the sooner the situation is recognised and supported effectively, the better it is for the learner as well as the supporting staff.

Let us consider other forms of disability that your learners may have.

Supporting learners with sensory impairment

Since the implementation of the Disability Discrimination Act in 2006, universities have had responsibility for accepting learners who have some form of disability. Normally, prior to acceptance, applicants to health care courses undergo an occupational health assessment as to their ability to fulfil the requirements of the programme and the relevant professional statutory organisation. Physiotherapy, for example, has led the way in accepting people with sensory impairment such as visual or auditory impairment.

Many learners who have a sensory impairment get tired much more quickly because of the level of intense concentration needed to adjust to the unfamiliar surroundings and to the activities taking place. In particular, people with visual impairment are likely to need more time to read or write up case notes, because of their need to read in a painstakingly linear fashion rather than getting the 'whole picture' by glancing over documents. They may also need longer to become familiar with the geography of an environment and with the people who work there because of the difficulty in recognising faces and shapes. However, many learners with sensory impairment have developed successful strategies to compensate for their impairment. In particular, they often have highly developed memory, communication skills, skills of analysis and problem-solving, planning and organisational skills. Vignette 5.4 describes how Claire, a 25-year-old physiotherapy learner who is partially sighted, can be helped to enjoy a successful placement.

Vignette 5.4 Physiotherapy learner, Claire, and her guide dog, Barney

Claire is in the second year of her physiotherapy degree course and is attending her second placement in the outpatient department of her local NHS Foundation Hospital. Her placements have taken place within easy distance of her home so that she did not need to use public transport or make unnecessary adjustments to her living arrangements. Claire had made a preliminary visit to her placement before starting so that she could become familiar with the route to the Department and so she could discuss her needs with the Practice Educator for the placement and to meet the staff. She also needed to make arrangements for her guide dog while she was working. Departmental staff had previous experience of supporting partially sighted learners and had taken advice from Guide Dogs for the Blind. To support Claire during her placement, they had provided a quiet corner in the physiotherapy treatment room for Barney, where he had his bed and a bowl for drinking-water. Staff knew that while Barney was wearing his harness, he was in working mode and should not be distracted.

Claire's visual impairment is not total, as she can see at a distance of 6m, but the objects are often blurred or indistinct. She has approximately 30% vision and is able to read large-sized fonts. To help her with her studies and while on placement, she has a small laptop computer to write her own notes and patient records, and a portable video magnifier, which helps her to read patients' notes. She also carries a digital recorder, which she uses to record verbal instructions about treatments.

During her placement, Claire will be mentored by Daniel, an experienced physiotherapist with previous experience of supporting partially sighted learners. He is aware that he needs to make an assessment of Claire's needs not only as part of his duty of care to assess her learning needs and her level of competence but also because he understands that sight impairment affects people in a wide range of ways.

After a shift of working together, they discuss the best kind of environmental modification that will help Claire. These include:

1. Using a designated cubicle – so that Claire will be familiar with where all the equipment is stored;
2. Having increased lighting to help Claire use her sight to the maximum and to ease her mobility without Barney at hand
3. Daniel encouraged Claire to talk to her patients and explain that she needed to make her assessment of their needs both verbally and by hand.
4. Specific equipment with tactile labelling would be kept in Claire's cubicle so she could use it safely once she had been supervised and seen to be safe.
5. The electronic notes of patients being treated by Claire and Daniel would be available in hard copy.

With Daniel's support, Claire was able to write up her case notes at the end of each treatment on her laptop and, using the wireless printer, could download and sign them before adding them to the patient's file.

Many of the principles used by Daniel to support Claire are relevant to other learners as well as to patients with sensory loss. An example is Katie is a 20-year-old midwifery learner who is deaf. Her mentor Alex is supporting her on her first placement in the ante-natal ward. Vignette 5.5 describes some of the adjustments that Katie might need.

Vignette 5.5   Katie, a first-year midwifery learner who is profoundly deaf

Katie is a 20-year-old midwifery learner attending her first clinical placement on an antenatal ward. She had made a preliminary visit to the ward with her link lecturer when they had met the manager and the practice education facilitator. In their discussion together, they had explored the kind of help that Katie would need during this first placement.

Being profoundly deaf since birth, Katie wore bilateral digital hearing aids and had her own digital stethoscope so that she could listen to blood-pressure and foetal-heart sounds. This had been the greatest concern for the clinical staff, since being able to listen was an essential diagnostic aid.

Having this preliminary meeting was reassuring for everyone involved, as Katie was able to demonstrate her ability to communicate effectively, and she felt reassured that the staff were willing to support her.

Point to ponder:

If you are Katie's mentor:

- What are your responsibilities towards your pregnant mothers, and how would you fulfil them?
- What are your responsibilities towards Katie as her mentor and as a representative of your employer?
- What other special adjustments might be needed in order to help Katie develop her midwifery skills during this placement?

Sometimes, wearing hearing aids does not help the deaf person, and they rely on lip-reading for communication. On some occasions, it might be reasonable and more cost-effective to provide a support worker as an assistant. The support worker will have been trained to undertake specific assistance activities such as translating verbal conversations to the learner using either sign language or lip reading. This may be helpful in settings where a profoundly deaf learner is working with people from a range of cultural and language environments, and so may have difficulty understanding their lip movements. Learners with sight impairment may also find it more effective to have a support worker to scan documents for key information requested by the learner or to translate diagrammatic or electronic information into written material, for example. At no time is the support worker used as a substitute for the learner, as their sole function is to improve the learner's access to the educational opportunities.

Supporting learners with mental-health needs

Government statistics indicate that approximately one in six of the population of the United Kingdom are suffering from a mental-health problem (NHS Choices 2012). They classify mental-health problems on a broad spectrum, ranging from anxiety and depression to the more enduring problems requiring life-time treatment such as eating disorders, substance addiction, schizophrenia and bipolar disorders. The Association for University and College Counselling (AUCC), which represents 530 counsellors and another 120 higher-education institutions, suggests that 3–10% of the learner population will have contact with its counselling service in a single year. With mental-health difficulties becoming increasingly prevelent in our society, it is likely that as a practice supervisor, you will encounter a colleague, or visiting learner, who is suffering from some form of mental-health problem. The kinds of disorders you are likely to encounter with visiting learners are problems such as anxiety, depression, substance addiction or an eating disorder. On some rare occasions, sufferers are admitted to their programme with the knowledge that they have a mental-health problem. As a result, they are able to receive the help that they need from the beginning of the programme and can enjoy their studies and be successful. More commonly, learners starting at university away from their home are plunged into an unfamiliar environment and encounter a range of challenges (such as the unexpected or traumatic death of a patient, verbal aggressiveness from a client and so on) that can lead to a sense of isolation and loss, causing anxiety or depression. In health and social care programmes, learners who are more likely to be faced with these kinds of challenging and uncomfortable experiences can easily slip into depression if they do not receive adequate support. These learners often experience a sense of isolation from fellow university students, who have little or no insight to, or sympathy for, their professional experiences. As a result of their feelings of loneliness, they may develop coping behaviours that may not be considered compatible with their professional status, while being common-place among other university learners.

Visiting learners need support when experiencing traumatic and alien events that resident staff may have come to terms with and found ways of rationalising or coping with successfully. Vignette 5.6 offers some insights and possible resources for a supervisor to use.

Vignette 5.6   Shona, a third-year radiotherapy and oncology learner

Shona has been allocated to the oncology unit for her penultimate placement. Martin, her supervisor was impressed by her general appearance and attention to detail. She had arrived in the unit at the start of a particularly busy week, and Martin had only time to show her around and show her what she could do, before having to dash off for meetings and treatments off site. Shona gave the impression of managing without her supervisor and of being generally very capable, although somewhat tetchy when other staff asked her to undertake particular (menial) tasks. The following week, Martin was on annual leave and had omitted to tell Shona this or who would be looking after her. When he returned from leave, he was dismayed to find that Shona's behaviour had changed, arriving late on duty and leaving early. She seemed withdrawn and uncommunicative, although none of the staff had discussed this with her.

What should Martin do?

Realising that Shona's behaviour was probably uncharacteristic and that he and his colleagues had let her down quite seriously, as well as breeching his Code of Professional practice by leaving her without supervision, Martin arranged for the two of them to have a meeting in a private place. At the meeting, Martin first acknowledged that Shona had been let down and apologised for not looking after her as well as he should have done. To his surprise, Shona burst into tears. Over the ensuing conversation, Shona revealed that she was having difficulty with her studies owing to family and housing problems. She is a single mother with three young children, one of whom goes to a day nursery, and the other two attend a local school. They live in rented accommodation, and her tenancy is coming to an end in four weeks' time, because the landlord is increasing the rent by 30%. She is desperate to find alternative housing and to finish the course so that she can start earning a salary. Over the past 3 months, she has lost 20 kg and is now seriously underweight; she is having difficulty sleeping at night and is unable to attend to her studies. She is also aware that she is being very irritable.

Martin recognises that Shona needs specialist help from the university counselling and learner-support services. With Shona's permission, he immediately contacts the radiotherapy clinical teacher and Shona's personal tutor, who come over to the unit to work out a plan of support with Shona. They help Shona make arrangements to see the counsellor later that day. The university counsellor and Shona agree a plan of regular meetings while she is going through these difficulties. With her help and through learner services, Shona is given emergency access to a family housing unit for university learners, which she and her family can move into while she is on her course, at a rent that she can afford with her learner grant.

Martin's relationship with Shona is now on a more collegial basis, and he recognises the importance of taking time to get to know his visiting learner at the very onset of their placement. He also acknowledges that he needs to be more conscientious in ensuring his learners receive support and appropriate supervision at all times, not only because of his duty of care to his patients and his colleagues, but also because learners are totally dependent upon their supervisor for their placement learning.

In Vignette 5.6, Shona is clearly a very capable person, having reached almost the end of her course while coping with very difficult and challenging social problems. It was clear that she had reached the end of her tether, and although she could not be labelled as having a 'mental-health problem', she was clearly suffering from a great deal of stress-induced anxiety and needed some professional help. It was fortunate that Martin had the maturity and the insight to recognise that he had made a mistake and that he had the courage to rectify it. As a result, Shona was able to resolve her crises and to progress towards a successful completion of her course. If Martin had not addressed the situation, it is probable that Shona's anxiety and stress would have caused her behaviour to become increasingly unsatisfactory, leading to a very different outcome.

Many visiting learners experience anxiety about starting a placement in an unfamiliar setting. Sometimes, this anxiety is made worse by academic difficulties or social problems. As a supervisor, you are in a good position to minimise such anxieties by taking time at the very start of their placement to get to know them and to give them the opportunity to talk about any support needs that they have. Vignette 5.1, where Gareth met his mentor and co-mentor, Mitch, on the first day, is an excellent example of how to prevent future difficulties and to give your learner the best chance to be successful. If your learner subsequently develops emotional or mental-health problems, your initial befriending will make it easier for her or him to talk about them, to receive help and to be successful.

Summary

In this chapter, we have explored the importance of making assessments of the practice of any new coming practitioner, whether it is a new colleague or a visiting learner. The aims of making such assessments are to fulfil your professional duty of care towards your clients/patients and your responsibilities towards visiting learners for ensuring they are able to make the most of the learning opportunities in your workplace.

Educational theories argue that people learn best when they feel valued and have some autonomy over their learning. You can promote their learning by making newcomers feel welcome to your community of practice, helping them to make informed choices about the learning opportunities that are available and by providing them with effective support and coaching.

Taking time to get to know your visiting learner also gives you the opportunity to learn about any support needs that they have. It is better if this information can be received prior to their starting the placement, as you may have to make adjustments to facilitate their learning. Legally, your organisation has a duty of care towards any learner or colleague who has a disability. It is very probable that your organisation has policies and strategies for preventing discrimination and for providing appropriate reasonable support. Reasonable support is intended to promote equality of access to experience during the placement that helps the learner to demonstrate their abilities. However, such adjustments are not intended to place them at an advantage over their able-bodied colleagues. Most of the adjustments that are agreed with the learner are simple modifications to everyday practice. Both professional statutory organisations and employers are required to provide training to staff who are likely to support people with disability as part of their continuing professional development. This may be provided by your occupational health department or by a designated disability officer. You can obtain support for your learner either from the educational representative in your organisation or through their personal professional tutor and the university learner services department.

Useful web sites for information

Disability support:

http://www.hse.gov.uk/disability/
http://www.delni.gov.uk/index/publications/pubs-das/das-employment-information.htm
http://www.rnib.org.uk
http://www.guidedogs.org.uk/
http://www.actiononhearingloss.org.uk/
http://www.bdadyslexia.org.uk
http://www.dyslexiaaction.org.uk
http://www.guidedogs.org.uk/

Mental-health support:

http://www.learnermentalhealth.org.uk/
http://www.learnerdepression.org

Chapter 6

Facilitating professional development

Jenny Spouse

Introduction

This chapter works with the concepts of a community of practice and learning as situated within a placement setting. It explores how learners might be introduced to the knowledge and expertise of the wide range of practitioners working in such a community. Using the lens of case studies or vignettes, we describe common practice placement situations to explore the kinds of knowledge pre-qualification learners identified as important to them. We shall also provide some snapshots of simple everyday activities that can afford significant learning and which can be easily adapted into your own practice.

Contemporary research studies into neurophysiology are influencing our understanding of how humans learn. These theories of learning are used to explore and to explain the snapshots and vignettes illustrating how you can best facilitate professional development through your everyday work and so provide rationale for your 'teaching'. Some of these vignettes will be reviewed through the framework of the Model of Practical Skill Performance (Bjørk 1999) and invite you to consider what additional information could have been shared. You may find this model of practical skills development a helpful tool to consider your own professional knowledge and to consider how you teach effective professional practice. You could also use this model to evaluate your learner's performance and thus their future learning needs. You may find it helpful to keep a journal of your own activities and to consider them against the ideas presented in this chapter.

This chapter includes the following:

- what learners want to know;
- learning to relate while working in a community of practice, exploring and explaining the learning;
- developing technical knowledge – the Model of Practical Skill Performance as a medium for promoting professional practice; vignettes and snapshots illustrating different kinds of teaching in a range of professional workplace settings – how to make learning opportunities; the learner as participator;
- legitimate peripheral participation; explaining and exploring social theories of learning;

Practice-Based Learning in Nursing, Health and Social Care: Mentorship, Facilitation and Supervision,
First Edition. Ian Scott and Jenny Spouse.
© 2013 John Wiley & Sons, Ltd. Published 2013 by John Wiley & Sons, Ltd.

- explaining and exploring: zone of proximal development, scaffolding learning: deciding, when and where to use learning opportunities;
- learning to bundle practice activities together – management skills;
- developing craft knowledge;
- managing personal feelings, developing the essence of professional practice;
- working in a community of practice; exploring and explaining the value of being welcomed: sponsorship, befriending, planning, confederation, coaching, flying solo and talking heads;
- summary of effective teaching, sharing of understanding and knowledge.

What learners want to know

In Chapter 5, we advocated that supervisors make an early assessment of their visiting learner's learning needs. You can make a preliminary assessment during your first introductory conversation, when you look at your learner's portfolio or learning passport (the document that is a record of their practice placement achievements and learning requirements) and discuss their aspirations. The next stage of assessment is the most critical and is when you actually observe what your learner can do currently and what s/he is capable of achieving during the placement. Such an assessment is aimed, not only as a means of planning future learning opportunities but is also an essential means to protecting your patients while fulfilling your professional obligations to protect the public (and thus your own professional registration).

In our discussion of supervising visiting learners, we will focus on how you can engage them in your everyday activities and those of your clinical team. We will not urge you to offer formal tutorials, because that is not your role. Instead, we explore the importance of encouraging learners to accompany you on your everyday tasks and the value of sharing (teaching) your professional knowledge, otherwise known as professional craft knowledge or fingertip knowledge. This is the kind of knowledge that you put into practice all the time and which learners are hungry to acquire.

Learners also need space to practise their new found knowledge but only when you are satisfied that they are capable and safe. Achievement of professional competence is complex and multi-faceted. In a study of nursing learners' professional development, Spouse (1998; 2003a, b) identified seven aspects of professional knowledge with which her research participants were concerned, each element providing a building block for the subsequent element (see Box 6.1). That these learners were able to develop skill in each element depended upon exposure to high standards of professional practice, opportunities to rehearse and refine

---

Box 6.1   Hierarchy of learning priorities in nursing (Spouse 1998).

Relating to patients and their carers
Developing technical knowledge
Bundling the tasks together
Developing craft knowledge
Managing personal feelings
Being therapeutic
Relating to and functioning within a clinical team

complex skills, and to develop understanding of the rationale for their actions. Although they have been presented as separate entities, in the ideal learning partnership, learners will have opportunities to develop each of them at the same time, and for the purposes of this chapter, we shall explore the first two: relating and developing technical knowledge.

Learning to relate to patients and their carers

During their early clinical placements learners are primarily concerned to understand how to relate to their clients/patients. They often have little experience of communicating with peers, adults or children as a professional. Sensitivity to their own inadequacy is increased when facing an unfamiliar and personally challenging situation such as caring for someone who is confused, facing death or for whom they have an inherent respect. Their classroom learning will have taught them the importance of developing effective inter-personal skills, but putting them into practice in the professional situation and especially when carrying out unfamiliar or complex technical tasks is challenging. Learners are often aware that patients are more likely to relax if they can talk to them while conducting a technical procedure but, because of their own need to focus on the task, often find it difficult to do so. To develop interpersonal skills, learners might use a simple task as an excuse to practise talking to their patients without feeling self-conscious. But in the early days of their placement, the more unfamiliar or technical the task, the more they need to concentrate on 'getting the procedure right', and the less emotional or intellectual space they have to engage in 'chit-chat'. Their self-consciousness is often heightened when being asked difficult questions by their patients, and so ensuring your learner has opportunities to watch skilled professionals undertaking this kind of work is invaluable (see Vignette 6.1).

Vignette 6.1   Anita's experience of learning to relate to a severely mentally ill patient

My mentor for this placement was one of the best I have had. Louise was really sensitive to her patients, giving the impression of being relaxed and focussed all the time. During the first week of my placement on the unit, I was frankly quite frightened about being there. Luckily, my mentor latched on to this, and she encouraged me to accompany her and to observe how she related to the patients. The first time we went into a patient's room, I sat in the background and just watched. Afterwards, Louise explained what she had been planning to achieve and why she had used the tone of voice and language. It was really helpful. We did this several times over my first week, mostly with her leading the way and me watching, but as I grew more familiar with how she worked, she let me have a go, and she would be the one sitting in the background. It was just a brilliant and reassuring experience. As the placement went on, we would still do this when there was going to be a tricky meeting with a patient or their relatives; she would let me sit in as well, so I could learn from watching her. I had classes on interpersonal relationships in Uni, and we had practised with each other, but seeing how Louise related to her patients made it all real for me and encouraged me to do more reading. When I was on my own and having to relate to patients, I found that I had an image of how Louise went about things in my mind, and it helped me when I was talking with them.

Anita is describing how her mentor, Louise, helped her to become confident in relating to their patients with mental-health problems. Louise provided a powerful learning experience for Anita by role modelling her actions. Humans are more likely to remember experiences when their emotions are involved. The stronger the emotion, the more vivid the memory, and thus the more enduring is the learning. You can probably recall some important experiences that have shaped your own practice as a result of your emotional response to a situation. In the vignette, Anita describes her apprehension when first working in her placement, so her memories of sitting in the background while her mentor talks to the client will be heightened by her strong feelings. Having opportunities to observe her mentor carry out the same activities several times, perhaps introducing nuances according to the needs of their individual clients, will help Anita retain the memories.

Exploring and explaining Vignette 6.1

Modern brain theory indicates that humans unconsciously learn from their environment (Damasio 1999), but because they are assimilating so much information all the time, they may not be aware that they are learning. Polanyi (1966) described this kind of learning, or acquisition of knowledge, as tacit knowledge. Some 'actual tacit knowledge' can be described, but more often it is impossible to find the appropriate language, and yet it is still possible to deliver a learned activity perfectly. It is possible that Anita's mentor, Louise, would find it very difficult to find the words to actually explain what she is doing when working with her clients, unless she has 'formalised' her actions by sitting down and writing about them. This is probably why so few practitioners appreciate the wealth of knowledge they are using in their everyday practice. It could also explain why learners find it hard to appreciate how much they have learned during their placements.

From this discussion, you can appreciate the importance of encouraging learners to accompany you in any aspect of your professional activity. Providing opportunities for learners to observe how you relate to your clients or patients is even more important when handling the more stressful and demanding encounters. People who are role models tend to offer solutions to problems the observer is experiencing and which they remember for future use, particularly if they see practitioners behaving in a manner that reflects their own values. As a result, they are more likely to assimilate the behaviour into existing knowledge patterns.

Jean Piaget (1896–1980), a profoundly influential Swiss biologist and psychologist, suggested that humans have an innate desire for equilibrium and achieve this by adjusting to their environment. Earlier chapters on the learning environment and how newcomers respond illustrate this. By adjusting to their intellectual and emotional environment, humans manipulate or modify their knowledge through the neural systems, described by Piaget as schema, used for storing it. Taking the example of Anita, from her academic studies, she will have learned about how to relate to a distressed client, so she has already developed a 'schema' or framework for storing such knowledge in her memory. From each new experience concerned with relating skills, Anita can assimilate into her existing 'schema' the knowledge gained (Piaget 1972) and so enlarge her schema, that is, her repertoire of knowledge (skills and understanding).

However, if Anita's first experiences of learning how to relate to clients with mental-health problems is contradicted by her subsequent studies and clinical experiences, she needs to adjust her thinking and to change her pre-existing schema. This process Piaget called 'accommodation' and is a more challenging process that may be resisted unless, as in this example, Anita is persuaded that the old knowledge and behaviour are inappropriate. If Anita is able to make the effort to understand and comes to accept her new knowledge, she will accommodate the intellectual changes it requires, and as a result her learning will be remain memorable. Achieving such a change in understanding can be difficult and painful, and is more likely when the learner is supported or is highly motivated to achieve a recognisable goal. Carl Rogers (1902–1987), the American psychotherapist and educationalist, recognised how difficult it is for humans to change their deeply held perspectives and described this as 'significant learning' that involves the whole person, their emotions as well as their sense of self (Rogers 1969). Another American, Jack Mezirow, an adult educator, described learning of this kind as transformative (Mezirow 2000). Transformative learning is often immensely challenging to the individual. Taylor's (1987) research into adult learners found that coping with unfamiliar and demanding academic work involves a series of stages, similar to those of grieving. Starting with a sense of personal discomfort and disorientation, the ultimately successful adult begins to identify and explore the cause of the problem until, through reflection and study, they can accept that their discomfort is not due to personal failure but because they are dealing with unfamiliar language and concepts. With such insights, they begin to share their understandings, and thus orientation and equilibrium is achieved.

The Russian psychologist, Lev Vygotsky (1978), came to similar conclusions, arguing that humans hold different understandings (knowledge), some of which are available for use, and some which need to be contextualised or helped to be activated. He described these kinds of knowledge with his model the Zone of Proximal Development. The inner boundaries of the Zone representing existing knowledge that is available to use and the knowledge that is in the Outer Zone and which is, as yet, difficult to articulate and to use because its relevance has not yet been recognised.

Current research into brain function seems to be confirming these earlier psychological theories. Studies in neurophysiology suggest that learning is an emotional as well as an intellectual activity. It also indicates that neural pathways need to be developed and firmly established for memory to be effective. So, with repeated exposure to new knowledge, we are more likely to retain the learning for future use. You can probably recognise that these theories have relevance not only to the social kinds of placement experiences described by Anita but also to those related to developing technical and 'purely intellectual' knowledge, which we go on now to discuss.

Developing technical knowledge

Traditionally technical skills are explained in terms of a procedure, that the correct sequence of actions is followed and that the process is conducted efficiently and safely. This behaviouristic approach to skill development suggests that a coherent and dextrous performance is as a result of much practice. Usually, learners have opportunities to practise in skill laboratories, where it is safe to make mistakes. Practising in a skills laboratory has fewer distractions than the busy clinical setting where vulnerable patients could be harmed by a simple error. Such opportunities help learners to overcome their cack-handedness and to develop their ability to use equipment comfortably. Technical skill becomes competence when learners are able to combine a range of additional and complementary skills with the technical task and the ability to make modifications to a procedure following accurate assessment of the situation in which they find themselves. Experienced practitioners are instinctively aware that skilled performance entails a more sophisticated approach and entails characteristics such as artistry and science in situations where the patient is the centre of attention and when their psychological and emotional needs are also acknowledged. Snapshot 6.1 illustrates how a seemingly simple task to an expert can be far more challenging to a novice.

Snapshot 6.1   Gwen's experience of walking a patient

I was working on my own for the shift, as my mentor was in charge. I needed to get a patient out of bed and help him to walk before leaving him to sit by his bed. The patient was 10 days post-op and wasn't mobilising very well. Before I started, I made sure that the chair and his gown and slippers were at hand, and that his bed was at a reasonable height. I explained what we needed to do and how I was going to help him, ensuring that he understood. But when we came to the actual procedure, I found it quite hard to help him move to the edge of the bed so he could get his legs over the side and put on his slippers and dressing gown, as he was really tense. This got worse as I persuaded him to put his feet on the round and to walk a few steps. Looking back on it, I realised he needed pain control, and his stiffness was because of his fear of pain. My mentor didn't like using pain assessment charts, but I think it could have been helpful here. – Gwen, first year of course

---

In this situation, Gwen knew the practical procedure for mobilising her patient. She had ensured the necessary equipment that she needed was at hand. She had conducted the procedure in a logical sequence, and it seems that she had given her patient all the appropriate information. Despite this careful preparation, she was aware that the procedure had discomforted her patient, making it difficult for him to cooperate or to benefit from the procedure. Gwen later realised that this was because his pain had not been adequately controlled. As a result, and despite her best intentions, Gwen (and her supervisor) had failed to provide a caring approach. This could be described as professional negligence on the part of her supervisor. Gwen was aware that there were tools available to assess pain management, but her mentor chose not to use them with the inevitable result.

Experienced practitioners are sometimes heard to complain that visiting learners do not want to do the 'basic' or essential tasks but want to take on the more 'senior' activities that they observe registered practitioners doing. Like Gwen, many novices have worked as an assistant practitioner prior to starting their professional programme and have probably learnt by trial and error many of the daily routine activities. They have probably come to think of themselves as competent and efficient. As a result, they believe they have all the knowledge and technical skills they need. They are unaware of how superficial their knowledge is and how ill equipped they are to practise as a professional. Many such learners struggle to recognise their learning need until they work alongside an expert practitioner. In their past role, they were probably expected to 'get on with it', with patients being treated as work objects to be completed within a specified time frame, irrespective of their personal needs. In their role as assistants, they lacked opportunities to learn about the artistry and science of their practice, why the care was delivered in a particular way or, more importantly, how to look at, and to listen to the patient or client knowledgeably. As a skilled and experienced practitioner, you can recognise a wide range of signs and symptoms from how the client is speaking, the subject and nature of their speech, whether they are breathless by the effort, whether they make eye contact, what their skin condition is like, how easily they can walk and so on. Giving novices opportunities to work alongside skilled practitioners gives them a range of learning opportunities, from managing apparently simple tasks to picking up tips that could be life-saving, in fact, learning a myriad of different and subtle skills that are the hallmark of an expert practitioner. Spouse (2003a, b) named this kind of close supervision 'Confederation', as it affords the learner opportunities to observe your actions and to acquire local vocabulary or the jargon of your clinical speciality. In this process of confederation, learners pick up the nuances of your practice, such as watching how you talk to clients, how you help them with their mobility, how you prepare and handle equipment and so on. Most practitioners take such activities for granted and have difficulty explaining to a novice what they do, and yet, as in Vignettes 6.1 and 6.2, both practitioner and learner benefit. Vignette 6.2 (Tessa) shows an example of how working alongside an experienced practitioner changed Tessa's belief that she knew 'it all'. Coming to this realisation was an important event in Tessa's learning and resulted from what Rogers (1969) and Mezirow (2000) call 'significant learning' or 'perspective transformation'. Tessa came to recognise that her old patterns of working were inappropriate and potentially harmful to her patients. She was able to acknowledge this partly as a result of her academic learning being confirmed by her observations and experience of working alongside a respected and effective professional practitioner. It was also due to Tessa's motivation to become a professional herself, and her willingness to learn from new experiences.

Vignette 6.2 Tessa

Tessa is in the first year of her BSC Nursing programme. Since the age of 16, she had worked in a local care home for older people. Her first clinical placement was on a rehabilitation unit for older people. During her first week, she shadowed Nancy, her mentor, and assisted in care delivery. This had involved assisting people with their personal hygiene and mobilisation as well as delivering a range of treatments including their medications. While they were working together, Nancy encouraged Tessa to practise her technical skills, and to learn how to combine them with observing her patients at the same time as talking to them. Tessa was able to see how to help patients with their mobility without causing them discomfort, how to help them enjoy their meal without feeling rushed and how to recognise a wide range of symptoms of health and illness. Nancy and Tessa would share their observations, thus increasing Tessa's professional vocabulary as well as her understanding of the different health care needs.

Over the next three weeks, Tessa delivered care to a small group of patients for whom Nancy was the primary carer. At the beginning of each shift, Tessa and Nancy would do a nursing round together and then discuss her plans for the shift. They would review this plan towards the end of the shift and agree the information that Tessa would write in the patients' care notes. Here are some of Tessa's thoughts on her experiences:

> I was really disappointed when I heard what my first placement was going to be, as I had so much experience of looking after old people before I started. I felt I just did not want to go back to that when there was so much more to learn. How wrong I was! Working with Nancy has been brilliant. She is so knowledgeable, and I really like the way she talks to the patients. I have learned so much! When I came on the ward, the staff said to me that I had a lot to un-learn, and it would be hard. I know what they mean now. I feel so bad about

the way I was looking after the people in the home, but no one taught me like Nancy has. I have picked up so much from working alongside her, all the little tips she tells me as well as the way she points out different things about the patients that I wouldn't have seen, like how one patient who has come in following a nasty scald to her legs, and they discovered that she has anaemia. She has a slight yellow tinge to her skin, and she has lost some of the sensation in her legs, and they found this is due to a vitamin B_{12} deficiency.

Vignette 6.2 describes how Tessa worked in confederation with her mentor, Nancy, a registered nurse. She encouraged Tessa to participate in the everyday care-delivery activities. As a result of this 'legitimate participation' with her mentor, Tessa has gained access to much of Nancy's professional or craft knowledge that she could not have learnt without such a close working partnership. Being given opportunities to deliver care that is important to the overall function of the placement gives Tessa legitimacy within the community of practice, helping her to feel that she is able to make a worthwhile contribution and that she is valued.

Because Nancy is concerned for the well-being of her patients and conscious of her own professional responsibilities, she continues to expect Tessa to work alongside her until she is satisfied that she is competent to work with more distant supervision. This is despite Tessa's rich background of experience in this area of nursing, although as a result of her experiences, Tessa is able to have her own tailored case load sooner than a learner with little or no prior nursing experience, but Tessa will still need support and supervision.

Explaining and exploring using the Model of Practical Skill Performance

The learners in these vignettes illustrate how difficult it can be to recognise the significance of what they see or do without support from a more experienced and knowledgeable practitioner. In Gwen's experience, she came to realise that although she had followed the procedure correctly, because her client had inadequate pain relief he was unable to cooperate effectively. Perhaps she came to understand this as a result of her own studies, or perhaps she worked with a more competent practitioner who ensured their patients were adequately prepared. In Tessa's account, she was able to witness an expert practitioner and to recognise the differences in approach to their patients and to the outcome of their actions. Both Gwen and Tessa gained insights into their practice that perhaps clarified some of their earlier academic studies and, as a result, experienced significant learning. Gwen had probably learnt from her studies about the importance of effective pain management as well as the principles of mobilisation. It was not until she found herself trying to put these principles into action and was frustrated by her failure that she came to associate her difficulties to a fairly simple but important omission. Reflecting on what had happened helped her to make the necessary links between theory and practice, and thus to benefit from a memorable lesson. Tessa's experience was much more profound and affected her whole approach to caring for older people, and so was more akin to a perspective transformation. She had lots of practical experience that contradicted her academic studies, and because her practice was her real-world, she believed that her approach was correct. It was not until she was confronted by the professional practice of a clinician who she respected that she recognised her faulty way of operating. Both these examples illustrate how what may appear to an expert to be fairly routine are in fact complex professional activities requiring significant skill and knowledge.

Norwegian nurse, Ida Bjørk (1999), developed her Model of Practical Skill Performance through her research into how novice learners performed essential tasks when nursing patients. She identified six elements to skilled performance (see Figure 6.1).

In her model, Bjørk (1999) identifies six components of competent practice, and this illustrates how simple tasks are in fact highly complex. Learners trying to become competent practitioners need support from expert practitioners to show them the different components and how to combine each of them fluently.

Substance refers to the inclusion of relevant content to the task at hand i.e. movement, instruction, information.
Sequence: The logical order in which the task is undertaken.
Accuracy: The correctness of the task activities.
Fluency: The ease & fluency in which the task is conducted, (i.e. planning & organisation)
Integration: Ability to manage a range of complex activities at once.
Caring conduct: Ability to tune into the patient's holistic needs by creating an atmosphere of patient centredness, respectful, accepting, encouraging & responsive

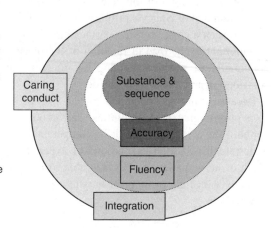

The circle symbolises unity & integration, with substance & sequence at the core. Each layer of the circle illustrates how every aspect of the action is related.

Figure 6.1   Model of practical skill performance (Bjørk 1999).

Legitimate peripheral participation

Legitimate peripheral participation describes the role that learners need to be given if they are to benefit from when working and learning in a busy placement. It entails providing your supervisee with a role that complements your own work. They have a workload that is important (legitimate) to the overall work of the team that is commensurate with their abilities and where they do not take the overall responsibility for the outcome (i.e. is peripheral). Of course, as a learner is assessed to be skilled and competent, it is beneficial to their progress to be encouraged to take on increasingly sophisticated workloads. But they continue to be considered learners until they have a professional qualification, and so supervision and responsibility for every aspect of their performance remain with their supervisor.

In Vignettes 6.1 and 6.2, we read how Tessa and Anita worked in confederation with their mentors. In legitimate peripheral participation, a novice may participate in a relatively minor or peripheral manner, such as assisting with bathing, or mobilisation, gradually increasing the level of participation until s/he is able to reverse roles with the supervisor (such as Nancy) who then assists and coaches rather than lead the delivery of care. As a result of providing legitimate opportunities for peripheral participation, Tessa (the learner) is able to develop her professional skills, partly from Nancy's coaching of technical activities (the substance, accuracy and fluency in Bjørk's terms), and with repeated experience of working with Nancy she comes to recognise how these tasks are integrated into an overall care package for their group of patients. By working alongside Nancy throughout their shifts in everyday care delivery and care-management activities, Tessa can pick up important snippets of information about their patients' medical and social history, and thus come to appreciate each patient's care pathway. She also comes to recognise Nancy's ability to be sensitive to her patients' emotional, physical and social needs by her interactions and her respectful and sympathetic approach: taking time to listen and to respond in a respectful and positive manner.

As a result, learning becomes an integral part of doing and thus more memorable and enjoyable.

In another situation, we see Gwen working on a surgical ward with a different supervisor, and together they are caring for a group of patients who have just returned from surgery (see Vignette 6.3).

Vignette 6.3   Working together – Gwen and Joy, her co-mentor

Gwen is working alongside Joy for the morning, and they are looking after five patients who returned from the surgical recovery room early that morning. Joy explains to Gwen that they need to make a nursing round of the patients to assess their condition. This involves introducing themselves to their patients, checking how they are feeling, so they can assess their mental state; then checking their physical status such as their vital signs, fluid balance, their wound and their pain control. In the process, Joy not only looks at the surface of the wound but also checks the bedding underneath each patient to see if there is any evidence of bleeding she might have missed otherwise. As they assess their patients, Joy chats to them explaining what she is doing, asking them if there is anything they need, perhaps a mouth wash, and explaining what she plans to do for them during the morning. This process takes approximately 30 min and has provided Joy with a huge amount of information, as well as reassuring her patients, reducing their anxiety and thus their pain. From the information gained, Joy can set her priorities for the shift as well as plan the morning.

Gwen has observed how smoothly and efficiently Joy works with each patient, helping them to sit more comfortably in their bed; giving them a mouth wash, or helping them to sip some water. In the process, Joy has encouraged them to practise their breathing and leg exercises to prevent complications. Gwen already knows how to read medication charts but needed practice in giving intramuscular analgesia. She has learnt what to look for when monitoring records of post-operative patients' vital signs and fluid balance. Joy has taught her not to take these obvious sources of information for granted but to make visual checks of the wound and the area behind it, as well as to observe her patients' condition by observing how easily they are talking and moving in their bed.

Having made their assessment and administered medications and fluids that are needed, Gwen spends the morning assisting Joy in delivery care. As they work together, Joy explains what she is doing and her rationale. When the third patient is comfortably sitting out of bed, Joy tells Gwen that it is her turn to lead the care delivery for the next two patients, and she will be Gwen's assistant. This experience gives Gwen a lot of encouragement, and she finds her confidence grows. In the process, she is putting into action what she has been observing Joy do. Towards the end of the shift, they discuss what they have been doing and how they will document their actions in the patients' records.

Points to ponder:

- To what extent to you think Gwen's partnership with Joy has helped her to develop professional knowledge as described by Bjørk's Model of Practical Skill Performance?
- During this shift, do you think Gwen has been able to observe any of the following kinds of professional knowledge: procedural, technical, interpersonal, scientific, aesthetic, managerial?
- Can you match the activities against any of the kinds of knowledge listed here?
- Are there any kinds of knowledge missing?
- How would you assess Joy's conduct against Bjørk's Model of Practical Skill Performance?
- What might prevent you from working with a learner in this fashion?

In this Vignette (6.3) and in Vignette 6.1, both Anita and Gwen were fortunate to have supervisors who were willing to have them 'on-board' throughout each shift. When Joy was satisfied that Gwen was going to be able to deliver care under her direct supervision, they reversed their roles. These examples illustrate how legitimate peripheral participation can be used in busy clinical settings. In Vignette 6.3, the learner (Gwen) is able to assist Joy in her work as a junior partner, and when the roles are reversed, not only does it give Gwen an immediate opportunity to practise what she has been learning, but also Joy can assess how much Gwen has learned and how safe it is for her to take on more responsibility with more distant supervision.

Explaining and exploring social theories of learning

Theories about how people learn have been mostly concerned with formal learning that takes place in the classroom or from reading texts. More recently, neurophysiology has provided tangible evidence of how we store and use knowledge. This understanding has led to a re-evaluation of educational psychology. Theorists have recognised that more learning takes place through everyday activities at home and in the workplace, and have tried to describe how this learning takes place. Leading this field of study is Russian psychologist, Lev Vygotsky (1896–1934). He disliked the experimental work conducted by his colleague, Pavlov, with animals and was more interested in the development and working of the human mind and speech. Through his research in the field, he theorised that learning was best achieved in the context of the subject matter through social interactions and facilitated what he called 'higher mental functions'. He also saw problem-solving (or learning) as a two-stage process, which he labelled the 'zone of proximal development' (ZPD; Vygotsky 1978). Vygotsky described the zone of proximal development as 'the difference between what a person can do independently (knowledge-in-use) and what they are capable of doing when guided to use their knowledge-in-waiting' (see Figure 6.2).

Vygotsky's concept of a ZPD acknowledges that people often know more than they can tell, in that their knowledge is waiting to be brought into use, or to be validated. You have probably discovered that learners often have some knowledge that they can talk about and enables them to function at a 'level' but, with probing or coaching, can bring into use what Spouse (2003b) describes as knowledge-in-waiting. You can appreciate what this means

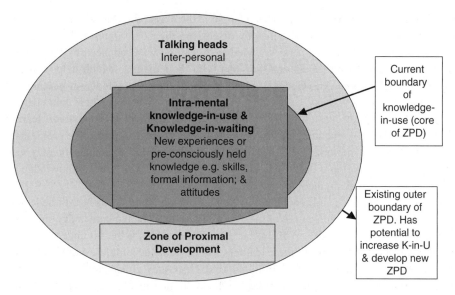

Figure 6.2   Zone of Proximal Development (adapted from Spouse 2003b).

if you consider how much visiting learners have studied prior to their clinical placement. They often arrive, having received considerable tuition both in theoretical material and in skills training, but they may have difficulty seeing the relevance of such knowledge to the patient before them, or to use it in their practice unless helped through coaching and 'sense making' with their mentor or their peers. Gwen, in Vignette 6.3, had learned about post-operative complications and the various signs to look out for. But not having been shown how to see them on real patients, she was unable to use her knowledge-in-waiting until Joy demonstrated how she brought such knowledge into use through her everyday practices.

If we use the analogy of a new bank debit card that is clearly identified as being for your personal use (it has your name, bank account number and a 16-digit identification number on one side and a security number on the other side), but the card will not work until you have validated it. The card is clearly visible but useless without an additional task made by you to activate it. The same is true of theoretical information and technical knowledge. It is not until the theoretical material is made relevant through discussion or by being put into practice that it becomes valid. With repeated exposure to the information and relevant practice, such knowledge becomes embedded in the memory, and learners are then able to use it more flexibly. They begin to recognise a wider range of circumstances where the knowledge is relevant, and to recognise more subtle differences, quickly. This is known as the theory of general principles, and as a result the knowledge can be used to solve increasingly complex problems.

Educational theorists, Marton and Säljö, described in 1976 (Marton and Säljö 1976a, b) how learners can be helped to develop their knowledge by relating new information to everyday experiences and situations. They named this way of acquiring knowledge a 'deep' approach to learning rather than a 'surface' approach used by learners who have rote-learned the information and can only recall facts. In Vignettes 6.1, 6.2 and 6.3, where learners worked alongside their mentor, we saw how Louise, Nancy and Joy encouraged their learners to bring what they had been taught in the classroom (knowledge-in-waiting) to use in their everyday care activities by discussing their care plans and care-delivery activities together. These learners' knowledge-in-waiting was enhanced by the 'talking-head' conversations and reflections they had with their mentor, which helped them to apply their classroom knowledge and thus bring their knowledge-in-waiting into knowledge-in-use. Vygotsky called these kinds of conversations, where knowledge is developed through discussion or by acting and thinking aloud, *inter-personal* learning (between people). By encouraging learners to use their knowledge to solve problems, to recognise clinical symptoms and to consider their cause and how to manage them, you are helping them to develop a deep approach to their learning, which links knowledge and experiences, thus making them memorable.

This kind of guidance and coaching illustrated in the vignettes shows how these learners were able to enlarge the inner core of their own ZPD and to change knowledge-in-waiting to become knowledge-in-use. With further practical experience but no understanding of its rationale or theoretical basis, these learners will probably accumulate more knowledge-in-waiting, but of a practical and attitudinal kind. Once they understand the rationale for their actions and are able to use their new skills in an intelligent and thoughtful manner, the knowledge becomes usable.

Having opportunities to discuss our observations with a more knowledgeable 'guide' is a valuable way to make sense of our experience and to learn from it. Vygotsky described this kind of talk between two or more individuals as 'inter-personal speech'. At other times, if no one else is available, and we need to guide ourselves through a complicated task for the first time, or when trying to work out a problem or when reflecting back on a day's work, we may talk ourself through the process. This kind of thinking aloud and reflecting while problem-solving Vygotsky called *intra-mental* (within the brain) speech, and both kinds of speech help us to develop higher mental functions. In Snapshot 6.2, Nick is using intra-mental speech to help him prepare for a procedure.

Snapshot 6.2   Nick's preparation for a procedure

Nick is preparing equipment for the house officer to set up an intravenous infusion for an elderly patient. The patient knows that the doctor will be coming at 4 pm to do this and is sitting comfortably in her bed. In the treatment room, Nick is working through the procedure and what will be required. He knows that it has to be an aseptic process to prevent the introduction of infection, and so the trolley needs to be spotlessly clean. He cleanses his hands thoroughly, and his intra-mental or personal speech goes something like this:

Well, the doctor'll need a dressing pack to prepare the skin site, with cleansing lotion. But he'll need to do this aseptically, so he needs sterile gloves and sterile lotion.

He needs an IV needle and giving set. Ah, but I need to prepare the set by running it through with normal saline. But that needs to be hanging up so that it flows, so I need a drip stand.

How is the needle going to be secured? I need some tape and a splint and a bandage to keep it in place. They can go under the top shelf of the trolley. Right, is there anything else? Oh, perhaps a fluid balance chart so the volumes of fluid going in and being excreted can be measured and recorded.

Clearly, Nick has some experience of seeing an infusion being set up and has a vision of what is going to take place, making it easier to get all the equipment prepared. In Snapshot 6.3, Anita is going to give an intramuscular injection for the first time.

Snapshot 6.3 Anita's administration of an injection intramuscularly

Anita has had some practice of giving intramuscular injections in the skills laboratory and with the simulator, but this will be her first time of doing it on a patient. She feels happy and confident when working with her mentor, Louise, and although she is apprehensive, she knows that she will be supported. Louise has chosen a slightly overweight patient to make this first injection less frightening for Anita to do.

Before they start the procedure, Louise asks Anita to talk her through what she plans to do (inter-personal/talking heads). Then, Anita starts by going to prepare the patient, collects the medication chart and returns to the treatment room. Talking herself through the process (intra-mental), Anita then starts the procedure, washing her hands first and collecting the required equipment. She checks the chart, collects the correct drug, checks it with Louise and, with a somewhat shaky hand, draws up the correct amount from the ampule and checks it with Louise. She explains to Louise what she plans to do next, and together they walk to the patient's bedside and go through the procedure to administer the drug, dispose of the needle and syringe safely, and complete the documentation.

Using talk in these ways, Anita is able to draw on her existing knowledge to think about what she needs to do and to apply her knowledge to her current situation. It will help her to recognise anything she has forgotten as well as to embed the knowledge more firmly in her memory.

Points to ponder:

- Thinking about a similar situation from your own experience, at a minimum what would you expect of Anita's performance if you were to describe it using Björk's model? (The six elements are: substance, sequence, accuracy, fluency, integration, caring conduct).
- How can you help a learner such as Anita to increase the quality of her performance?
- Why do you think it is relevant for Anita to feel confident with her mentor, Louise?

Exploring and explaining: scaffolding and coaching

A follower of Vygotsky, American educational psychologist, Jerome Bruner, and his colleagues described scaffolding as an activity when we learn from being guided or coached by another, more knowledgeable person or by talking ourselves through the activity (Wood et al. 1976). In Vignette 6.1, Anita's mental-health placement, her mentor encouraged her to observe her skilled interactions with mentally ill patients and then arranged her workload to include opportunities to practise these relational skills. The opportunity to observe Louise provided Anita with a 'scaffolded' experience that helped her to see how her own prior learning (about interpersonal skills and relating to people with mental-health problems) was being implemented in the clinical situation. Louise provided further scaffolding by discussing her actions and encouraging Anita to 'have a go' with suitable patients. In Snapshot 6.3, Louise again provided scaffolding to help Anita develop her technical skill in administering a drug by injection. At the same time, it is probable that Louise used the opportunity to help Anita extend and apply her knowledge of pharmacology as it related to this patient: the reasons for the drug to be given, its actions and side effects.

In Vignettes 6.2 and 6.3, both Tessa and Gwen had mentors who also used scaffolding techniques such as planning legitimate work activities that were relevant and that promoted their learning. They worked in a confederation partnership followed by taking on leading the care under their mentor's direct supervision and coaching.

Following activities as illustrated in these Vignettes, for example, with discussion or 'talking heads', such as talking through the procedure, debriefing and reflective practice, also provide a scaffold to their learners' development of knowledge from knowledge-in-waiting to knowledge-in-use. Table 6.1 illustrates how these three learners were provided with scaffolded learning experiences and demonstrates the different ways in which you can promote learning.

In these three very different examples, we can see how each of the learners gained from their experiences of working alongside an experienced practitioner and extended their knowledge, both practical and intellectual.

Anita had no prior experience of relating to people who have a mental-health illness, but by observing her mentor, Louise, and then being able to discuss her observations with her mentor, she was able to develop some mental models of how she would like to relate, which increased her confidence.

By contrast, Tessa had a great deal of practical experience, but because previously, she had no effective supervision despite her good intentions, she developed inappropriate practices and attitudes to older people. It is not until Tessa works alongside an experienced practitioner that she realises there is a different and more attractive way of operating. Gwen in Vignette 6.3, on the other hand, when she is starting surgical nursing, is being given close support and supervision. As a result, she learns how to develop competence in caring for acutely ill patients.

Bjørk's Model of Practical Skill Performance provides a useful means for thinking about your own practice as well as providing a framework for assessing your learner's progress. Each aspect of the model makes explicit quite complex and sophisticated actions that, as a practitioner, you may not be conscious of. As a supervisor, you could use the different elements of the model to discuss your own practice, your aim being to help your learner to integrate a range of sophisticated professional skills, the technical and theoretical knowledge, the interpersonal, the organisational and the time management skills, and to learn how to use such knowledge in their practice. At the same time, you are giving them the opportunity to make a valued and legitimate contribution to your overall workload.

Learning to bundle practice activities together

An essential skill of practitioners is the ability to manage a case load of clients. Even novice learners need to work out how to plan and prioritise their actions. Bjørk's Model of Practical Skill Performance has two components concerned with organisation of work: sequence and fluency. Sequency is concerned with ensuring the detailed steps of the action are performed in a logical order, while fluency is concerned with combining each aspect of the performance in a smooth manner. For novices, it is a

Table 6.1 Scaffolding learning – three learners' experiences.

Stage	Anita's experience	Action: inter-personal scaffolding
1	Anita had some theoretical knowledge as well as life experience of interpersonal relationships, but not with people who were mentally ill, and was uncomfortable with them	Anita recognised that she felt uncomfortable about relating to people who were unpredictable and was able to talk about this with her mentor, whom she respected
2	Anita was actively involved with Louise, her mentor, who encouraged Anita to observe how she practised an activity that is taken for granted by expert practitioners in mental health	Being able to observe her mentor in action, how she responded to different and challenging situations, enabled Anita to accumulate a repertoire of techniques that she then tried out with patients herself
3	Anita recognised the relationship between some of the literature and her clinical observations, and wrote a reflective account of her experience and increased confidence	Anita's reflections on her experience both with her mentor and in her reflective account enlarged her ZPD, bringing knowledge-in-waiting to knowledge-in-use through both inter-personal and intra-mental scaffolding

	Tessa's experience	Action: inter-personal scaffolding
1	Tessa has extensive practical experience of delivering essential care to older people as a care assistant. Inadvertently, her actions are often brusque, poorly sequenced, lack substance and accuracy.	Tessa participates in care delivery with Nancy, an experienced geriatric-trained RN who 'talks aloud' when helping patients ambulate
2	Tessa is impressed by the fluency of Nancy's thoughtful actions. She finds she is learning new ways of acting, practically and emotionally.	Nancy's care illustrates an approach that dignifies her patients and gives them a level of autonomy. She also explains the rationale for her actions that are fluent, integrated and demonstrate a caring comportment.
3	Tessa has learned a great deal from participating in care delivery with Nancy and is incorporating her learning as best she can when delivering care	

	Gwen's experience	Actions: inter-personal scaffolding
1	Gwen is new to a surgical ward and is learning how to deliver care to new post-operative patients	Gwen participates in a nursing round of her mentor's patients. Together, they make an assessment of their patients' physical and emotional well-being and decide their care-delivery priorities.
2	Learning how to conduct a physical assessment: what signs and symptoms to look out for; how to assess fluid balance status; how to assess pain levels, how to incorporate preventative measures in her care	Gwen watches her mentor as she checks different areas of the wound site and as she monitors the patients' levels of hydration and pain. Her mentor explains her actions and reasons while she is doing them and encourages Gwen to fill in the documents.

(continued)

Table 6.1   *(cont'd)*

3	Practice at administering intramuscular injections	Having identified pain-management needs, Joy supervises Gwen as she administers the drugs
4	Practice in delivering care to new post-operative patients	Gwen assists her mentor in essential hygiene and mobilisation techniques and delivers preventative care. Their roles are reversed for two patients, and Gwen is the lead care giver supported by Joy.
5	How to manage a group of patients, to set priorities, organise oneself and to exhibit skilled practical performance	By watching how Joy organised herself, the kinds of conversations she had with their patients and how fluently she conducted the various technical skills, Gwen was able to recognise high-quality care being delivered

challenge to manage care delivery to one patient without forgetting some vital piece of equipment or being interrupted by the patient who has a greater need, such as pain relief or the need to use the toilet.

As learners progress through their placement and develop the necessary essential skills, they can take on a larger case-load and thus further develop existing skills. Part of Gwen's experiences with her mentor, Joy, in Vignette 6.3, was witnessing how Joy planned and organised her care. Gwen learnt the value of first assessing the needs of their group of patients, ensuring they were in a fit condition to receive the care, assembling the necessary tools and delivering the care without unnecessary interruptions. Managing a group of patients is more complex than managing care delivery to one patient, so it is important that you give your learner opportunities to acquire these skills. As you become satisfied that your learners are safe to practise under more distant supervision, you can give them opportunities to deliver care to a group of patients. This often increases their confidence and motivation to learn, as Snapshot 6.4 illustrates.

Snapshot 6.4   Marie and her case load

I have been on the placement four weeks, and I am feeling that I am really getting into it. My mentor has given me half of her case load for the shift, and at the start we planned what I would do and the order in which I would deliver the care. Now that she knows I can do it, she leaves me to get on and make my plans alone. I have enjoyed it so much because I feel that I am learning all the time. Before I get off duty, I go and read up about the people I am looking after the next day and so I know what to do. So, I am learning about their different conditions and their treatments, which is really good. If I have a problem, I know I can ask my mentor for help. At the end of the shift, we discuss what I have been doing and what I will write up in their records. This gives her some feedback as well as helping me to learn what I need to say.

In this snapshot, Marie describes how her mentor has taught her to plan her workload, to set her priorities and to evaluate the effectiveness of the management plan. Having a preliminary conversation with your learner helps you to feel confident about what they will be doing and that your patients will be safely cared for. The process also helps your learner to justify their plans (inter-personal scaffolding) and to recognise any potential pitfalls that can now be avoided. The end-of-shift discussion again helps you to identify any omissions so that they can be dealt with quickly to avoid any problems. The debriefing process of talking about their actions is another inter-personal scaffolding activity, which helps your learner to gain insights while they review their plans and to think about managing their case load differently. Giving your learner opportunities to discuss their practice also helps them to gain a deeper understanding of what they are undertaking. As Snapshot 6.4 illustrates, Marie was so excited about being trusted to have her own case load that she felt motivated to find out as much as she could about their condition and how best to look after them. Through this process, she was able to increase her ZPD by the intra-mental scaffolding of studying, thinking and planning.

Being able to delegate a case load of patients to learners is also helpful to you, as it provides some mental space for your own well-being as well as more time to attend to some of the other demands on your time.

Developing craft knowledge

Professional craft knowledge is the kind of know-how that experienced practitioners use without a second thought. They seem to have the know-how at their fingertips and are able to anticipate difficulties and how to prevent them or to manage tricky situations without having to worry. Patricia Benner, applying research by the Dreyfus brothers (Dreyfus et al. 2009), described how post-qualification nursing practitioners can develop their capability by learning from experience and progress from being a novice to becoming an expert. The core element of their progress is developing their professional craft knowledge.

Many learners are unable to bring their classroom knowledge into use when in practice. Classroom knowledge inevitably tends to be generalised from everyday practice rather than be specific to an individual or a situation. As a result, learners need help to see how their classroom knowledge relates to what is before them. In Gwen's case (Vignette 6.3), her mentor was talking her through the assessment activities she was doing and showing Gwen the difference between a normal set of observations and an abnormal set. It is likely that she asked Gwen to explain why a patient who is haemorrhaging might have a raised pulse, lowered blood pressure and be sweating, all symptoms of deepening haemorrhagic shock. It is probable that Gwen would have been able to explain, but would not have recognised the symptoms without her mentor's support.

For many learners, it was not until they have acquired a level of confidence to think beyond the technical aspects of practice that they began to actively seek out formal knowledge to inform their practice (as Marie describes in Snapshot 6.4). Spouse's small study of nursing learners (Spouse 1998) suggested that learners needed to reconceptualise themselves as nurses (i.e., that they could function in a legitimate role within the community of practice) before they had the mental space to think about how to explain their actions or the underlying theory. Once learners felt competent in everyday technical skills, they could relax and were more able to function within the clinical team. Then, they could begin to make connections between what they were experiencing in their practice and what they had learned either in school or from their reading. Over time, they could then develop their practice towards the element described by Bjørk as 'caring conduct'. This is where the practitioner is able to combine every element of an activity (substance, sequencing, accuracy, fluency and integration of all these aspects) in a manner that communicates respect, compassion and support to their patients in a knowledgeable way.

Benner et al. (1996) suggested that expert practitioners appear to have a repertoire of solutions to different problems that they can tap into as the need arises. This implies that once learners have achieved a level of capability in technical skills, they need opportunities to work alongside a range of different practitioners in the same clinical environment so they can see how different practitioners manage the same or similar situations. This helps learners to develop their own repertoire of professional craft knowledge.

Managing personal feelings

Many learners begin their professional career with a personal vision of how they would like to relate to their patients (Spouse 2000) and use this image to inform their everyday relationships. Often, such images are also coloured by perceptions of how they 'ought' to behave as a professional. Questions such as, 'Is it alright to cry when something sad or joyous happens?' and 'How should I behave when a patient or a relative is consciously rude towards me, or when someone makes a sexist or racist remark?' Learners are often caught in a dilemma, as they are taught to be authentic in their behaviour, and yet there seem to be some situations where it is inappropriate to respond from the heart, such as when personally attacked either verbally or physically. Having opportunities to observe how an experienced professional deals with such situations is helpful, but sometimes even such observations can create personal conflict. Snapshot 6.5 provides an example where Harry is learning how to relate to adults who are struggling with everyday activities.

Snapshot 6.5　Harry witnesses his mentor using humour

At first, I thought it was inappropriate for my mentor to make jokes with the patients. But they didn't seem to mind, and it distracted them from their frustration at not being able to get dressed as quickly as they wanted. It also helped them to relax. When I read up about using humour in practice for my reflective journal, I realised that when used appropriately, it is an important inter-personal skill. Psychotherapists such as Rogers (1961) argue that therapists should be honest in their relationships and so using humour if it is suitable in such situations then it is OK.

Points to ponder:

- What kind of learning was Harry engaging in here?
- Was this kind of dialogue inter-personal dialogue or intra-mental?
- How does this approach to delivering care fit into the model of practical skill development?

In this vignette, Harry has witnessed his experienced mentor use a strategy that he found uncomfortable, as he was afraid she might be perceived as laughing at her patient rather than with him. Through his reading, he came to recognise that this was a deliberate action designed to distract her patient from his frustrations at not being able to move. As a result, Harry decided to keep the strategy in his repertoire and to try it out when working with similar situations.

Another major challenge for learners is how to respond to patients or relatives who ask questions that they find difficult, particularly about dying. A learner will be aware of the prognosis and the policy of how much information is divulged. Unless they are supported by their mentor, they are unlikely to know how to deal with such questions or indeed whether they should respond. If you are aware that a situation such as this might arise, it is helpful to provide some guidance to your learner about how to respond and, even better, to provide an example by role-modelling how you help a patient in such a situation.

It is very unlikely that learners have peer support in their lodgings to discuss how they should behave, and often they are left on their own to worry about it. In a related situation, Shirley, in Snapshot 6.6, feels isolated by the lack of communication from her colleagues.

Snapshot 6.6 Shirley and the empty bed

I had a placement on the unit for six or seven weeks and knew all the patients there quite well. There was one older lady who was a wonderful character, very strong-willed and determined to go home once she could walk with a frame. I came up to give a group of patients their treatment after a few days off and found that she was not there, and her bed was occupied by someone else. I asked the staff whether she had been discharged, and they told me she had died two nights previously. I was so shocked that I didn't know what to do or to say. I just felt awful and wanted to get out of the place and cry. The staff appeared to be indifferent, and seemed very hardened. It was awful. I just wasn't expecting it.

Points to ponder:

- When Shirley was given her workload at handover, should the staff member have warned her about this patient's death?
- What support could Shirley be given when receiving this news?
- Are there any support services in your organisation that could help someone like Shirley who is experiencing bereavement?
- Bjørk's Model of Practical Skill Performance could also apply to how this clinical setting was being managed – to what extent was caring conduct demonstrated towards Shirley?

Smith's work (Smith 1992) indicates that the emotional style of the person in charge has a strong influence on the quality of care – the caring comportment. Shirley's experience suggests that the staff she talked to either had repressed their own feelings, and so had forgotten how others may feel, or were indifferent. Hochschild (2003), writing about air hostesses and debt collectors, first described 'Feeling Rules'. These rules relate to situations when there is a conflict of emotions, and to deal with it people, such as health social care workers, put on 'a good face. It may not be appropriate for them to express personal feelings in a public situation, but it is essential for their feelings and actions to appear to be congruent. Unless they can find ways of coping with such situations, they are likely to suffer stress and even burnout (Smith & Lorentzon 2008). In supporting your learner through emotionally challenging situations, it is helpful to acknowledge that your work is emotionally demanding and to encourage discussion and to share your own strategies for coping.

Another aspect of emotional work that learners struggle with is to find a means of navigating through the range of ethical dilemmas that they experience. Issues concerned with people who have a terminal illness, or who experience heroic treatments, are particular worries. Other concerns are associated with delivering care according to plan, such as encouraging people to eat and drink when they are either too confused or too ill to want to accept the care; encouraging mobilisation or prevention of complications when the person has insufficient pain relief or fails to respond to pain management treatment. More subtle dilemmas are frequently associated with observing how colleagues contravene good practice by talking over an individual or gossiping about one; see Snapshot 6.7.

Snapshot 6.7   Tessa's concern

Tessa was working with a new health care assistant (HCA) on a medical ward. They are nursing an elderly man who has suffered a stroke and is not yet conscious. While they work together, Tessa is upset that the HCA is rather rough with him and is spending the whole time gossiping about her friends and family, and does not seem to be concerned about the patient. Tessa is aware that he might be able to hear what is being said and might be upset by some of the conversation. She tries to suggest that they should talk about something else, but the HCA dismisses her suggestions and carries on chatting.

Tessa wonders how she should have managed the situation and whether she should speak to her mentor.

Points to ponder:

- As a mentor, what opportunities do you provide for your learner to talk to you about such experiences?
- What kind of responsibility does Tessa's mentor have towards this patient and are there any actions to be taken?
- Do you think the HCA needs any help or guidance and, if you do, what?

Developing the essence of professional practice: therapeutic action – caring comportment

Most of the vignettes and snapshots that we have presented illustrate situations where learners are anxious to develop a high standard of professional practice. They are concerned about the quality of their technical competence as well as the other elements that make up skilled performance. As they become more capable and confident, they also become aware of a further aspect of their practice that is concerned with being therapeutic. Jourard (1971) describes nursing as a public form of loving that promotes self-development of the practitioner by their learning to be open, honest and in touch with the 'self'.

Developing such self-knowledge when faced with the challenges of a demanding professional course and exposure to failure can be intensely difficult and painful, unless supported by the same kinds of care from their mentors and supervisors. Watson (2009) describes the importance of nurses nurturing their colleagues and themselves if they are truly to be able to provide care. Bjørk's Model of Practical Skill Performance provides a model for developing caring skills that you may find useful to guide your own mentoring practice when supporting a learner.

Working in a community of practice

Learners often worry about wasting their mentors' time, having recognised the huge workload that they are often managing. They feel guilty at taking up their time without having a means to reciprocate in some way.

In earlier chapters, we have introduced the phrase 'Community of Practice' to describe a group of people working towards the same aims. The group may be located in the same geographical environment such as a clinic or a ward; alternatively, individual community of practice members may be engaged in the same clinical speciality but working in different geographical locations across the world. Through social media, they can share their ideas and developments, thus learning and developing their practice from using the network as an educational and social community. These practitioners may for example all work in the same profession such as radiography or nursing or be a multi-professional group working in a specific area of practice such as care of older people, cancer care or a specialist practice such as substance abuse in mental health or in renal medicine. You are probably already aware of the many different professional fora, journals, conferences and web sites for specific professional interests and may be using one of the web-based sites for increasing your professional understanding. For the purposes of this chapter, we have considered your workplace as a community of practice to which newcomers (novices, visiting learners or new staff) come to gain professional knowledge in your specialist practice.

Research by educational anthropologist, Jean Lave, and psychologist, Etienne Wenger (Lave & Wenger 1991), and their colleagues investigated learning in traditional communities, and from it we have the term 'community of practice'. Their research and that of subsequent educational anthropologists have become increasingly helpful to describe learning in the workplace. Their findings also confirm earlier work by Russian psychologist, Lev Vygotsky, and his followers, including educationalist, Jerom e Brunner. Current theories of learning by contemporary theorists argue that learning is most effective in the social context (see, for example, Illeris 2009), and from their research, we can identify five fundamental principles of learning in a social setting or a community of practice:

1   people are social beings and so gain their identity from their social environment;
2   people learn best in a social setting;
3   learning increases as the newcomer acquires the vocabulary of the community and knowledge of the everyday tasks they are undertaking;
4   learning takes place when the newcomer is encouraged to participate in tasks at a level commensurate with their ability;
5   designated tasks must be relevant to the overall work of the community of practice.

Busy practitioners sometimes find it difficult to know how to manage their already huge workloads along with supervising learners. They may misunderstand what is meant by self-directed learning and feel that their role is more like a sign-post (Spouse 2001) or a facilitator, rather than an active educator. Vignette 6.4 provides an example of what happens to a learner who is not sponsored into a community of practice.

Vignette 6.4   Katy and mentor, Mike

Katy is in her second year and has been allocated to an adolescent mental-health ward for her specialist placement experience. She has been worried about this placement, as it is very different from her experiences of nursing young children, her last placement. She had gone through the usual preliminary procedures prior to starting. When she arrived on the ward, it was clear that the place was very busy with a lot of noise and people rushing around, ignoring her. She managed to collar one of the nursing staff in the office and introduce herself. This person clearly didn't know who she was; neither was he expecting her. Katy was told to sit in the patients' sitting room, and her mentor would come and collect her. After waiting for an hour, Katy decided to have another go at finding her mentor, who was on duty and, as it turned out, was sitting in the coffee room having a drink. Katy introduced herself and explained what had happened. Her mentor, Mike, apologised and invited her to have a chat over a coffee with him. He then suggested that she went to talk to a couple of the patients while he gave out some drugs and attended to some treatments. Although feeling she was being abandoned yet again, Katy felt she needed to make a good impression and found the two adolescents. By the end of the shift, Mike still had not returned, and it was clear that he had forgotten about her and had even gone off to his lunch. By this time, Katy was feeling completely disheartened and wondered what the rest of her placement was going to be like. She decided that instead of giving up, she needed to have a chat with the practice-educator to see if she could have a different placement supervisor who was less busy.

Points to ponder:

- What do you think Katy should have done about this experience?
- What might have happened to Katy if she had been more assertive and refused to be left in the patients' sitting room, or again if she had refused to be 'dumped yet again' when she was told to go and talk to the two patients?
- What do you think the practice educator might do about the situation?
- If the situation is not resolved satisfactorily, what might happen to Katy?
- To what extent was Katy admitted to the community of practice and given sponsorship?

  From the Mentor's perspective:

- What preparation could Mike have made for Katy?
- How could Mike have involved Katy in his daily work?
- How should Mike resolve the situation and fulfil his responsibilities?

In this vignette, we are describing a fairly common experience for many learners. You may have a similar story to tell. In this vignette, it is possible that Mike might have misunderstood his role as mentor and did not know about sponsorship. He might have felt that he was encouraging Katy to be self-reliant and self-directing, and he might have decided that she was failing to match up to these expectations by not taking the initiative. You may feel that Mike's behaviour, although understandable in a pressurised working environment, is not appropriate. Indeed, there is an increasing volume of literature indicating that learners are often treated badly, such as being ignored or physically isolated, verbally abused or receiving negative comments about career choice. Such experiences are described as vertical violence (see, for example, Lewis 2006; Thomas & Burk 2009). Many learners are so disillusioned by their treatment by people they had expected to be role models and exemplars of their profession that they leave their course (see Spouse 2003b: 77).

In the example in Vignette 6.4, it is quite possible that Katy will feel so disillusioned and unwelcome that she will leave as soon as she can, if she is a new member of staff. If she is a learner, making such a choice poses significant dilemmas and raises a number of difficult questions such as: Does this mean she will be seen as a failure? Is it the end of her aspirations? Who is available to help her? If there is a clinician or an academic able to support her, can she be given an alternative placement or mentor?

In our discussions about effective learning environments in Chapter 3 and again in Chapter 5, we argued that the most crucial factor in any setting is the quality of the social environment. This is particularly important for newcomers, either new colleagues or visiting learners. Having someone who is willing to take responsibility for inducting the newcomer to the setting, providing sponsorship, gives them a greater sense of security and frees up energy to take notice of what is going on and to engage in the general activities of the social group, rather than being pre-occupied and worried (Spouse 2003b). With effective sponsorship, the newcomer is reassured and feels welcomed, and so has the intellectual space to remember facts, vocabulary and activities that might otherwise be forgotten or unnoticed. If the sponsor (such as Mike in Vignette 6.4) is unable to have the visiting learner work alongside until he or she is competent and safe to function independently, then it is crucial that another, appropriate, member of the community of practice is delegated to chaperone/supervise and teach the learner. Without this kind of close supervision, you could be putting your patients at risk as well as jeopardising your visiting learner's future. You could also be jeopardising your own career. It is as serious as that.

Most health and social care professions stipulate that their qualified practitioners have a duty of care towards the public, and so they are personally accountable if this duty of care is breached, even if the 'injury' is caused by another person who is under your supervision.

In Vignette 6.4, it is possible that if Mike had known about the importance of sponsorship, he might have made some preparation for Katy's arrival by reducing his workload for the shift and ensuring he could spend it with Katy. He could have involved her in his daily activities giving her the role of a legitimate participator. He could have taken her along with him when he was dispensing the various medications as well as letting her shadow him in his other work. At the end of the shift, they could have discussed his work and planned her next shift. By doing these simple activities, Mike would have helped Katy feel welcomed, rather than feeling she was in the way. He could have provided a role model for Katy to see how to relate to adolescents with mental-health problems, and at the same time observed how she was interacting with their patients and so making a preliminary assessment of her capabilities.

Exploring and explaining the value of being welcomed to an unfamiliar social environment

Several theorists (Dewey 1939; Vygotsky 1978; Belenky et al. 1986; Brunner 1987; Jarvis 2009) argue that people gain their identity from their social environment and that personal development is achieved through social interactions. Jarvis (2009) suggests that even in the womb, the foetus is acquiring knowledge, even if unable to articulate what it is, later in life. Jarvis supports Dewey's argument that by engaging in everyday practices, and thus by immersion in experience, we become sensitive to patterns of activities and, with the development of vocabulary, can construct meaning from them. Learning, he argues, is through both body and mind; our physical and emotional experiences of life are often more powerful than the intellectual experience (Jarvis 2009).

Research into how nursing learners learn by sociologists such as Simpson (1967) and Melia (1981) found that learners adopted the practices of their nursing peers when working in clinical settings, even if it contradicted what they had been taught in university. Like Tessa when working as a care assistant described in Vignette 6.2; they believed that the learners used this strategy because to do otherwise exposed them to rejection and was consequently too emotionally painful. To be 'different' meant they were more likely to be rejected or embarrassed by their perceived ignorance or by their inability to use the same vocabulary, to meet the same workload expectations as their community of practice peers. Alternatively if they believed the inherent practices of the placement staff contradicted their learning they may be brave enough to question (or challenge) inherent attitudes and practices and thus suffer rejection. For learners in Simpson and in Melia's studies their success in the placement was vitally important, and so they were even more anxious to become socially accepted. Learners in these studies complied with the norms of their placement community and, as a result, were more likely to be accepted and thus given learning opportunities. Once established or accepted by peers, they found it was possible to modify their personal behaviour so that it was congruent with their personal beliefs. If learners find compliance too difficult, they are more likely to leave their course or the job (see Spouse 2003b: 77).

A study by Jordan (1989) of Latin American traditional midwives describes how they were required by their government to attend a course on western obstetrics in order to continue as midwives in their home community. During the course, they appeared to comply with the philosophy and practices of the course and so were successful in completing it. But on their return home, they did not utilise their learning of western midwifery because the beliefs conflicted profoundly with their own personal beliefs and those of their community. These traditional midwives had moved from one culture to another and then returned to their home culture. To survive the course, they needed to adapt their identity. On return to their own community, they re-affirmed their identity to match the values of their traditional community which held quite different beliefs about conception, birth and the role of the midwife. Adapting to the values of each specific community of practice was more important to their survival and thus to their livelihood.

Wenger, having explored learning in traditional societies, then investigated learning in commercial settings and developed a model. This model describes his theory of learning in the social environment (Wenger 1998). In his model, he identifies four elements that

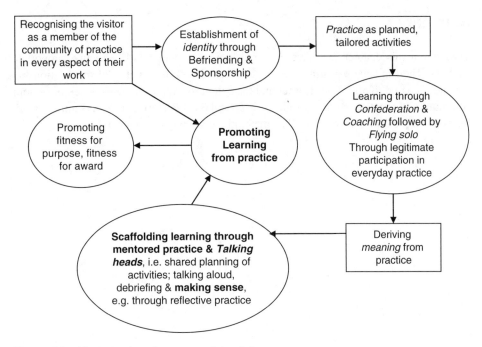

Figure 6.3 Mentoring learning as a social activity.

influence learning: *identity, community, practice* and *meaning*. Spouse modified this model to explain findings from her research investigating how nursing learners developed their professional knowledge (see Figure 6.3).

This model illustrates the importance of the four stages in effective mentorship: *befriending* – welcoming the newcomer to the placement and helping them to feel part of the team; *planning* an itinerary for learning; *confederation and coaching* practice – a two-stage process where the newcomer works alongside you as 'lead' practitioner, and when you know your learner is sufficiently capable, the roles are reversed, with the learner leading the care delivery under your supervision and coaching. This is followed by flying solo, when you give your learner a case load under distant supervision; *Talking heads* entails you and your learner discussing the issues at hand, such as helping your learner to plan their work, setting priorities, discussing their intended actions, listening and supporting them while they talk themself through their actions, discussing ethical or practical issues and so on. Talking heads also includes creating opportunities for your learner to discuss their actions afterwards, thus encouraging them to reflect on their actions. This is often a good way to help them acquire the vocabulary of your community of practice as well as helping them recognise the significance of actions. It is a way of preparing them for writing their reports and documenting their actions. Another way of helping learners develop meaning from their practice is by encouraging them to write up their practice activities using relevant literature thus helping them to take a deep approach to learning and to develop a wider understanding of their work.

Summary

Throughout this chapter, we have explored how you can provide effective support to learners. The fundamental principles are concerned with the quality of the relationship you are prepared to offer your learner and the extent to which s/he feels welcome at your community of practice. Bjørk's Model of Practical Skill Performance offers a framework for assessing learning needs as well as the kinds of knowledge you can share.

Chapter 7

Reporting on progress: assessing performance and keeping evidence

Ian Scott

Introduction

This chapter looks at a variety of methods that you can use to assess the skills knowledge and capability of your learners as well as yourself. Assessment is fundamental to the role of the facilitator and is likened to two sides of a coin. On one side, findings from assessment indicate what needs to be learned, and on the other side, it indicates how successful that learning has been.

By reading this chapter, you will gain a better understanding of different types of assessment and when to deploy them, what to assess, how to assess and what makes a good assessment tool. In this chapter, we also review the difficult subject of failing learners and suggest some different ways to improve your abilities as an assessor.

This chapter includes the following:

- the nature of assessment;
- different forms of assessment;
- assessment as learning;
- the learner's perspective on being assessed;
- deciding on criteria;
- making the decision, knowing what is being assessed and coming to judgements;
- failing students;
- improving your assessing.

Assessing and assessment

Being able to assess the skills, knowledge and capabilities of learners is a key activity for anyone who helps to educate others. If you are unable or unwilling to assess a learner, you will not be able to help determine their learning needs or what your learner has achieved, or to assess the effectiveness of the learning strategies that you used. Assessment is complex, has many facets and is certainly contentious. The Quality Assurance Agency for Higher Education (QAA) in the United Kingdom discusses the reliability and validity of

Practice-Based Learning in Nursing, Health and Social Care: Mentorship, Facilitation and Supervision,
First Edition. Ian Scott and Jenny Spouse.
© 2013 John Wiley & Sons, Ltd. Published 2013 by John Wiley & Sons, Ltd.

assessments as an area of concern throughout their reviews of different subjects taught in higher-education institutions (cycle 1993–2001; QAA 2003). In the National Student Survey (NSS), a survey open to all finalist Higher Education learners in the United Kingdom, assessment and feedback have consistently been given the lowest satisfaction ratings of any of the elements of the survey areas since the NSS's inception in 2005.

Assessment is a natural process through which every human being gathers information. The information is used as a means against which to judge people or situations using pre-established criteria. These criteria are not necessarily written or spoken and are most often held internally to us. Think for example of how you choose a holiday destination, how you judge whether a situation is risky or how you came to decisions about talking to a stranger. These types of decisions often rely on previous experiences, and we often use our intuition to judge new situations against past experience. Rowntree (1977: 4) describes assessment as a process that occurs 'whenever one, in some kind of interaction … is conscious of obtaining and interpreting information about that person'. Assessment of learning is an extension of this process with the distinction that we try to make sure that the criteria against which we are making judgements are explicit. One definition of assessment taken from the University of Oregon Teaching Effectiveness Program defines assessment in the context of education as the following: 'Assessment is the process of gathering and discussing information from multiple and diverse sources in order to develop a deep understanding of what learners know, understand, and can do with their knowledge as a result of their educational experiences.'

Point to ponder:

• In relation to your clients/patients, how do you make judgements about their needs?

In relation to learners in health or social care settings, assessment needs to occur as soon as possible, so your clients are not put at risk by the practice of an inexperienced professional or a learner. You are no doubt only too well aware that if someone under your supervision makes an error, you are responsible, both ethically and in the eyes of your profession and the law. Bearing this in mind illustrates the importance of making early and ongoing assessments of your supervisee's capability before delegating any aspect of their workload.

Types of assessment

Formative assessment

Formative assessment is a means of telling the facilitator and their learner about their existing level of capability and knowledge. It can also be used to assess what progress has been achieved during a period of practice. Formative assessment indicates learning needs and provides information about the effectiveness of the strategies you are using to help your learner achieve competence and whether or not these strategies need to be adapted or changed. Formative assessment should thus be designed to maximise learning, help to build on strengths and to identify areas that need more practice or focused development.

In Chapter 5, we discussed how useful formative assessment can be to identify your learner's needs and how this assessment can be used to plan their placement experiences. Using assessment in this manner helps your learner to feel valued and to feel that their learning needs are being taken seriously.

Formative assessment is often described as ipsative in nature. This means that the assessor uses evidence taken from the learner's earlier performance and looks for improvement relative to that previous level of capability rather than with reference to any externally imposed criteria. Formative assessment in health or social care situations tends to be much more iterative and discursive than summative assessment. Formative assessment is 'low stakes'. It should not be of consequence to a learner's professional progression if they do not do well in relation to one or more aspects of formative assessment. The formative assessment should provide a platform for acknowledging achievements and launching forward to establish how future progress can be sustained and achieved. Effective formative assessment relies on the use of regular feedback and of that feedback being delivered expertly. We shall be discussing how to give feedback on Chapter 8.

If you are providing mentorship or supervision that is not part of a formal programme that leads to a qualification, it is likely that all the assessment that you do will be formative.

Points to ponder:
Take some time to consider when you last felt that you were being assessed.

- How did you feel?
- Was it important to you to succeed?
- Have you ever assessed someone else's learning?
- What do you think they were feeling and how might this have influenced their learning?

Summative assessment

Within the context of programmes for the qualification of new professionals, there will be times when assessment is formal and documented. In most cases, it will be referred to as summative assessment. Summative assessment is assessment that is designed to 'sum up' what has been learnt during a period of learning; it normally involves the formulation of judgements as to the quality and quantity of the learning that has taken place. Judgements often come in the form of grades, marks or pass/fail decisions. While summative assessments can be used by learners to help them obtain information on the progress of their learning and future needs, and can be used to evaluate the effectiveness of the learning strategies used, the main purpose of summative assessment is to make judgements.

As a matter of expediency in many professional training programmes, the role of mentor/supervisor and the role of summative assessor have been rolled into one. Unfortunately, this can lead to tensions within the relationship between the learner and the facilitator. Some argue that it is difficult to see how a developmental, supporting, empathetic relation can grow, when there is the spectre of 'critical judgement' hanging over the relationship. On the other hand, where a relationship does become close, how then can an objective judgement be made? In 2010, the Nursing Times published a survey of 2000 mentors that found 37% of the sample admitted to passing nursing learners practice, despite their concerns about their level of competence or attitude, or despite thinking the student should be failed. One of the interpretations of these findings was that mentors were reluctant to fail learners, as they believed it would reflect badly on their teaching abilities.

Summative assessment has a very strong influence over how learners prioritise their learning. They believe that summative assessments indicate what is important to know and do and what can be ignored. If you are a student and short of time, you are more likely to focus on those things that are critical to your success, and these will be those things against which a judgement is being made. The phenomenon of learners being assessment-driven is not new and certainly not confined to poor learners. Gibbs and Simpson (2004–2005), in their work identifying conditions under which assessment supports learners' learning, noted several studies indicating the great extent to which learners at top universities across the world were assessment-driven. Many authors have also noted that changing the nature of an assessment can affect the way individual learners engage with their learning. Thus, the design of assessment processes, particularly summative assessment, is of crucial importance. It is therefore crucially important that mentors and supervisors play an active role in designing summative assessments for practice learning.

Informal and formal assessment

Given our earlier arguments that assessment is a natural process, it is clear that not all assessment, even in the context of education, will be obvious and formal. It is unlikely that whenever you are observing your learner, you are going to be shouting out 'Here comes another assessment!'. In fact, quite the contrary: much assessment is actually informal, and after working with your learner, you may simply say 'You did that well' or 'You gained that client's respect'. Indeed, you may not have been actually aware that you were assessing. This type of assessment is informal assessment. Its informal nature means that it can be used much more developmentally or strategically. For example, you can use informal assessment as a way to challenge your learner beyond what is required by the formal assessment criteria. During informal assessment, you may observe something that, while safe, was not 'quite' as it should be, allowing you to decide whether to mention the point to your learner and to choose the moment to do so.

It stands to reason that all summative assessment will be formal, while formative assessment can be either formal or informal. You may have noticed that we used the word 'should' in the last sentence, because there is an important exception to this that considerably muddies the water. This type of assessment is continuous assessment.

Continuous assessment

Continuous assessment is not a new idea; in fact it probably dates back to the early apprenticeships of the middle ages that we discussed in Chapter 1. The concept behind continuous assessment is relatively straightforward. It is that rather than wait until the end of a period of learning for a judgement to be made, judgements are made continuously and that all these judgements are brought together to arrive at an overall consideration of the individual's learning. Continuous assessment seeks to combine the developmental aspects of formative assessment with the 'meaning' and significance brought by high stakes summative assessment. In relation to assessment in practice areas, it also means that a student cannot just 'perform' for the summative aspects; they must continuously demonstrate capability as assessment if de facto is continuous.

By contrast, the downside to continuous assessment is that it is not always clear to learners when they are actually being assessed, or what is being assessed. It means that no assessment is really ever informal and can sometimes give rise to learners presenting a façade hiding the capability they really have. Continuous assessment can also be argued to lead to more tensions in the facilitator/learner relationship particularly where a friendship as well as a professional relationship occurs. Nevertheless, continuous assessment is one of the most commonly occurring forms of assessment in practice-based education.

Points to ponder:

- In your practice area, which type of assessment (formative, summative, continuous) do you think is appropriate for the types of learning that you facilitate?
- Why do you think this type is appropriate?
- What issues can you see with this approach to assessing practice?
- What type of assessment do you believe your learners prefer?

Some assessment principles

Assessment in some form or another is an essential part of the process of professional development. When the assessment is informal and even done by ourselves on ourselves (self-assessment), there are certain ideas that underpin, or at least should underpin, all assessment, and these are discussed below.

What to measure?

Yorke (2011) suggested that when assessing professionals, we should be looking for three types of what he termed 'achievement': what knowledge, understanding, values and capabilities the person can demonstrate:

- as they engage in their professional work;
- in the way s/he goes about her/his work;
- through achievements in work situations.

For the purposes of this chapter, we have reversed the order in Yorke's (2011) original paper for the last two items. This is because we view the last item as a complex function of the first two items. The first item represents the 'tools' the individual has with which to do the job; the second item represents how those tools are applied; and the third item reflects the results of those applications when applied in the right combination and at the right time.

The blending of these kinds of achievement indicates, as Eraut (2010) is at pains to point out, how complex professional behaviour is.

Criteria

Criteria form the basis against which we make judgements (assessments). Behind this simple statement, however, there is hidden significant complexity. In theory, it should be possible, when looking at an element of practice, to describe how that practice 'should be', including the actions that make it complete and how the actions need to be completed in order for it to be correct. We may also be able to describe actions that can make that practice badly performed, and Bjørk's model (1999) described in Chapter 6 illustrates areas of practice for consideration. For example, when undertaking an action for a client, criteria concerned with interpersonal skills may include whether consent was gained or whether the practitioner introduced her- or himself when interacting with a new patient or client.

As you can imagine, professional practice is so complex that it is hard to describe all the nuances and variables that make up a particular action. I am sure that you have come across wide variations in the practice of your fellow professionals, but can you really describe all the aspects of the excellent practitioner that distinguish them from the 'just OK' practitioner? One problem with criteria that emerges from this discussion is that many of the criteria we use to make judgements are known to us and probably other experienced professionals, but they are tacit. They are taken for granted and are not discussed, and so often remain unspoken and internal to each one of us alone. Using these tacit criteria, we recognise good practice when we see it, but describing it in precise detail is very difficult. New professionals tend to learn about these hidden criteria through their experiences of working with a range of other professionals and developing their own repertoire of tacitly understood criteria. Working with these hidden criteria is normal and often workable within mentoring/supervision relations that do not involve formal assessment. However, in formal systems of assessment, using tacitly held and 'unspoken' criteria is no longer acceptable, for, if there are no criteria, how does the learner know by what standards and expectations they are being judged? This becomes a significant problem when it comes to distinguishing between learners in different stages of their professional programme and their development. Several professional authorities have developed standards of performance or criteria for assessing learners. Nicol et al. (1996) devised a frame work for assessing clinical and communication skills that followed the American nurse researcher, Patricia Benner's (1984) model of skill acquisition. Using this model, they believed it was possible to produce criteria schedules for specific areas of practice for differing levels of individual development. Table 7.1 illustrates one such schedule for communication skills below. It is described at three different levels: mastery, competent and foundation level.

Points to ponder:

- Looking at the criteria described above, would they help you to make assessment decisions?
- How do you think these criteria could be improved?
- Can you imagine any unforeseen consequences of your potential improvements?

This continuing problem of lack of clarity has led many curriculum planners for professional courses to outline very detailed standards and in some cases criteria against which candidates should be judged. This detailing of criteria is probably seen at its most

Table 7.1 Levels of competence in communication (Nichol et al. 1996).

Skill mastery	Competent performance	Foundation level
Communication skills are a natural part of every professional interaction Cognitive: affective and psychomotor components are highly developed and less subject to interference from other ongoing activities Performance based on increasing knowledge and experience: is confident, efficient and responsive to situational cues Reflection is central to practice at this level Safe and accurate performance with indirect supervision in the care setting The student is able to use an appropriate blend of communication skills, in a coordinated and effective manner The student is aware of his or her limitations and seeks help and advice as appropriate The student is able to adapt his or her performance in response to changes in the care situation	Safe and accurate performance under direct supervision in the care setting The student is able to utilise and blend communication skills together The communication skills chosen are appropriate to the patient/client and the situation The skills are executed smoothly and appear natural The student is aware of his or her limitations and seeks help and advice as appropriate The student is able to adapt his or her performance in response to changes in the care situation Safe and accurate performance with indirect supervision in the care setting The student is able to use an appropriate blend of communication skills, in a coordinated and effective manner	The student is able to identify the rationale for use of the skill but tends to reiterate textbook explanations The student is able to state when use of the skill is appropriate, and to what degree Performance of the skill is awkward, and the student may appear self-conscious

extreme in relation to National Vocational Qualifications (NVQ) introduced into the United Kingdom in 1986. These NVQ criteria were designed as a means to improve the standard of vocational qualifications. NVQs were designed on the assumption that all the 'activities' within a particular vocation could be identified, and a standard of performance could be written for each with criteria for assessing achievement of each standard. Box 7.1 lists some of the criteria for an NVQ in Health. Note that these are just a few criteria from a single unit; an entire NVQ is composed of several individual units (City and Guilds 2005).

These 'Criteria' are also supported by a range of statements in relation to the knowledge that a candidate should achieve in order to be able to demonstrate competence. In other words, the NVQ embraces the notion that 'being able to do' on its own is not enough.

Box 7.1   Sample criteria for NVQ in health.

Operate within the limits of your own role and responsibilities with regard to health and
    safety
Seek additional support to resolve Health and Safety problems where necessary
Use appropriate methods and procedures when taking potentially hazardous work
Ensure that appropriate people know where you are at all times

---

Point to ponder:

- Take one of these criteria and note down the evidence that you would want a learner to demonstrate before you could say that they had met the criteria.

The NVQ system has many detractors; for example, Knight and Yorke (2003: 210) suggested that as standards and criteria gain greater specificity, they start to exclude many practices and lead to 'the entangling and disorientating jungle of details as was experienced by those faced with the system of NVQs'. In addition, it is claimed by others that such bureaucratic systems to measure competence often fail to capture the 'essence of good practice' (Eraut 2003: 3). Perhaps surprisingly, research suggests that even when practitioners such as mentors and supervisors are supplied with detailed criteria on how to assess, in reality they do not use them.

Yet for us, perhaps the greatest issue with the type of criteria described above is that although they seem to be quite specific when assessors use these very precise terms, they always find them quite hazy (Knight and Yorke 2003). Their intended meaning only becomes clear when facilitators, tutors and learners interpret them, which does not guarantee that the criteria are being used uniformly by all assessors. In professional contexts when a learner's future is being decided, we need to work on ways in which we have a shared understanding, and this can only come about through dialogue.

For learners, this means that written criteria alone will always fail to encompass what is really being assessed, and it is quite common for them to feel unsure about 'what the assessor is after' and 'what they are looking for'. Failing to realise this is often a source of great frustration. In practical placement situations where learners are exposed to their mentor's practice, it is vitally important that the standards required for assessment are being role-modelled.

Competence

Professional qualifications emerged as a way to protect people from incompetent charlatans. Thus, it seems logical to assume that those practitioners who determine which learners should be professionals should be able to define competence. As a mentor or supervisor in health or social care practice, you are assessing the competence of your supervisee. To assess competence, you will probably be using standards to help you make judgements.

When we described the use of NVQs, we referred to standards. This term 'standard' emanates from the world of engineering and refers to a performance requirement of a component of system. Thus, in terms of human performance, a standard refers to the basic level of performance or ability that someone must be able to demonstrate in order to be an effective part of a system. So, it is humans that define the standard, and it is the community of practitioners that determine what this standard looks like in practice. Often, the term 'competence' is used synonymously for the term standard. Indeed, the Nursing and Midwifery Council in the mid-2000s switched to using the term standards from competencies to describe the abilities expected of nurses and midwives applying for professional registration.

The notion of competence, thus, seems like a straightforward concept, but because we need to describe the 'competence' in words, and they are bounded by context, finding a definition is not as straightforward as it may seem. To illustrate this, we use an example of competence based on a hypothetical carpentry course described by Scott (2011) below:

> 'Bang a nail into a plank of wood without splitting the wood'. At first glance, this seems like a straightforward competence, and very useful if you are a carpenter, but the carpenter who may employ the student might ask: 'Which type of wood' or 'which type of nail?' So, I would need to moderate the competence so that it might become, 'Bang the appropriate nail into a plank from a range of commonly used timbers without splitting the wood.' Of course, after speaking again with the qualified carpenter, she thinks that accuracy is also important and of course safety and this does not seem to be included. We are then confronted by the carpenter from the ship yard, who notes that what is a common wood for some is not common for him, how was he meant to tell what I meant or what these student carpenters were meant to learn.

The issue illustrated by this example is not easy to solve. What it illustrates is that the context in which discussions take place about the meaning of a particular competency statement needs to be discussed with learners and other professionals.

Eraut (2003) also raised some issues with the notion of competence. In particular, he raised questions concerning whether competence for an individual was constant or context-related and influenced by time and space. We can ask the following questions, for instance:

- Does our competence remain the same for example throughout a 12 h shift; or does it change between the start of the week and the end?
- If we qualified in setting X, are we competent when we move to new setting Y?
- Does our competence change depending on the expectations of our clients and workplace?

In essence, Eraut (2003) asked whether competence is individually or socially situated. When competence is considered to be individually situated, it is something that belongs to an individual and is transferable to different situations. When competence is considered to be socially situated, competence is shaped by the relationship between the individual, the context in which they work and, to some extent, the society that they serve. In this latter definition, competence is much less transferable and is changeable. Consider, for example, the snapshot of Natasha's experiences (Snapshot 7.1):

Snapshot 7.1   Natasha's competency when changing placements

Natasha has been a first-placement learner on a care of the elderly medical ward that spe-cialises in treating people with Alzheimer's disease. Most of the patients have long-term chronic conditions requiring a range of different medications. By the end of her placement, Natasha has become competent in communicating with her patients and has learned a great deal about the complications of polypharmacy. Her mentor has been most impressed with her ability to function as a junior member of the team, including taking a small case load. All the staff are sad to see her leave. After a week on her new placement, an acute orthopaedic surgical ward, Natasha is feeling completely demoralised and bewildered. The difference in expectations of staff is profound, and Natasha is feeling a failure.

Points to ponder:

- Why do you think Natasha might be feeling such a failure when she seems to have been excellent in her previous placement?
- As Natasha's mentor, what can you do to reassure her?

Eraut (2003) defines competence as 'being able to perform at the expected standard', noting, however, that the standard will vary depending on circumstance and the commu-nity's expectation. In Natasha's case, it is clear that her move to the surgical ward has had a profound effect on her self-confidence. She can see that she is not functioning at the same level of competence as she was on her first placement. If we accept what Eraut (2003) is telling us, it is predictable that Natasha would struggle until she has adjusted to this very unfamiliar environment and has learned some different skills as well as to adapt those skills she had acquired earlier. We can appreciate that competence is not a static phenomenon and is not something that one either has or does not have but is developed and modified according to the setting in which we are working. As an assessor, it is vital that you are able to appreciate this important fact. It is useful to consider the concept of competence as being 'dynamic' in terms of professional development. If we consider professionals developing through a programme of education, it becomes reasonable to have different levels of expected competence as learners progress through their pro-gramme. Furthermore, it allows us to recognise that their level of competence will vary depending on where they have been working previously and the requirements of the new setting. It will also vary depending upon the quality and level of support they received in the past and are receiving in the new placement.

Conversely, however, contextually defined competence causes an assessment conun-drum because poor performance may not in fact be linked directly to an individual's actual capability. It could be linked to a range of factors, for example, the quality of the team, the equipment available, the systems of support, whether individuals feel they have responsibility and accountability for their workload, and the quality of team communication.

Points to ponder:

- What factors might influence your competence as a mentor.
- How might changing your work location alter your competence?

Consider, for example, the case of Baby 'P'. Baby 'P' was a 17-month-old toddler who was abused by his parents throughout his short life. Before he died, it was known that he had suffered at least 50 injuries over an 8-month period (Campbell et al. 2008). His death caused widespread concern across the United Kingdom and much criticism of the handling of his case by the local authority concerned, which was Haringey Council. The various inquiries into the Baby 'P' case highlight how a combination of poor individual levels of competence and a disabling context ultimately led to the inability of the health and social services to protect this child from his parents. One of the criticisms of the social workers concerned was they lacked competence in that they were too ready to believe the parents' story and did not remove Baby 'P' from his parents' care. The cultural context to this story is also important to consider. Prior to publicity surrounding this case, there had been other similar situations that had been subject to an inquiry. Following the subsequent recommendations, social workers had been encouraged to do as much as they could to keep vulnerable children in their parents' care and that removal was to be considered only as a last resort (The Lord Laming 2009).

- What might be the impact of public expectations on the competencies expected of social workers?
- Can you give an example to support your conclusion?
- Do you have another example from a different profession?
- Will you have the same expectations when assessing the competence of your learner as a result of reading this section?

Learning outcome

If you are helping with the education of learners in collaboration with a higher education partner or are studying on a higher-education course, you will probably have come across the term 'learning outcome'. The learning outcome in higher education developed from outcome-based education within the vocational sector and is a relatively new concept in this context. A learning outcome is a description of what a learner will have learnt at the end of a period of study. Learning outcomes in theory can encapsulate a wide range of knowledge types, skills and behaviours. We can thus have learning outcomes that describe: particular skills, such as operating a microscope; ways of thinking, such as analysing; ways of behaving, such as respecting clients; and the possession (de novo) of good old fashioned declarative knowledge (knowledge and understanding that is accepted as fact by the wider world). In some settings, learning outcomes are also written in relation to the values that the learner needs to be able to demonstrate (e.g., valuing inclusivity).

The pedagogic purposes of learning outcomes are clear, in that they are designed to give a clear indication of the learning destiny that the learning opportunity provider intends the learner to reach. In doing so, they give power to the learner, since, armed with knowledge of the destiny, the learner can if they wish chart their own journey to this destination. It is this potential for empowerment that allows the proponents of outcome-based education to claim that it is 'student-centred' and is in contrast to the previous model where often the learning goals were perceived to be hidden, and known to the teacher only. Curriculum models that use learning outcomes, as logic would dictate, try to ensure that assessments test that learners have reached the destination described by the learning outcomes.

A further development to this is seen in the constructive alignment model of Biggs (1996). In this model, the totality of the curriculum and assessment is aligned with the learning outcomes. Indeed, it is Biggs's model that underpins much of the quality assurance system in UK education. The learning outcome is used to define the level of learning (Davies 2000), and differing scales of opportunity, for example at the level of the individual session, unit or course.

To the potential learner, a learning outcome describes what will be learnt; to the potential employer, they describe what should have been learnt; to the quality agencies, they provide a system for audit; and for the funders (if there are still any left), they provide a means to account for how their money was spent.

The learning outcome, as with the notion or criteria and standards, is a temptingly simple concept (James 2005). It seems to do exactly what it says it does, but unfortunately learning outcomes suffer from all the issues of culture, context and language (Scott 2011) that we have described above under the discussion of criteria.

Doing the assessing

Our discussion so far sets the scene for making an assessment. Even if you are not involved in a formal assessment of your learner, you will still be concerned with assessing their performance. This helps you to monitor their progress and to make useful interventions to support their development. As you will have read in Chapters 5 and 6, assessment always involves some form of observation. This observation can be either direct observation, such as when you actually watch the person you are mentoring or facilitating, or indirect observation, where perhaps you listen to the observations of others or the accounts of your learner. You are probably in the habit of assessing a situation before you undertake any interventions, and perhaps it is such a habitual activity that you are no longer aware of making the assessment. Thus, it is also reasonable to make an assessment of your learner before they engage in practice. You can make your assessment by exploring their relevant knowledge or perhaps by 'running' them through a simulation of the anticipated practice. As a mentor or facilitator, you are quite often concerned with assessing practice as it happens, but it is important to ascertain the level of supervision that your learner requires to be safe, before they start to work with your clients.

Assessment methods before 'real' practice can include items such as the following (adapted from Yorke 2011):

* performance during simulations;
* analysis and reflection on the performance of self and others during simulations;
* review and reflection of past performance;
* discussion of practice prior to practice;
* discussion of case studies;
* engagement with client case discussions;
* challenge scenarios;

- assignments and tests through which professional knowledge and understanding can be assessed;
- testimonial of witnesses to past performance.

Points to ponder:

- Can you find any other approaches to add to this list?
- If you were a student, how might you feel about being assessed by each of these methods?
- Which of these methods of assessment might you add to your repertoire of mentoring skills?

Use of these assessment methods will enable you to get a very good idea of your learner's current level of practice. These methods also present exciting opportunities where you can facilitate learning. You need to decide the criteria that will inform your decision before making a judgement of your learner's ability using these methods. Your criteria should preferably be transparent and, where possible, be agreed and discussed with your colleagues and your learners; in other words, you all need to agree, to some extent, on what precisely is being assessed and what you are looking for. Assessments during real practice could be based on activities such as the following (adapted from Yorke 2011):

- direct observation of learner by the mentor (which could involve checklists);
- direct observation of practice by another professional;
- direct observation of practice by a service user;
- direct observation of group activities;
- discussion of practice as it occurs;
- observation of practice through 'new media' such as digital video or voice recordings.

Notice how it is difficult to get away from the conclusion that the only way to assess practice in action is by being there, or relying on another 'trusted individual' to be there. Assessment that comes after a 'real' practice activity will always be indirect but includes:

- reflective analyses or commentaries (e.g., diaries, essays, documenting/recording work);
- debriefs with mentor/facilitator;
- reviews of practice decisions;
- challenges to rationalise and explain practice;
- reports on professional activity and achievements (e.g., workplacement).

Your choice of assessment method needs to be linked to the type of activity and the environment that your learner is practising. Sometimes, for example, when your learner is being assessed, carrying out a client consultation and obtaining consent may be difficult. Other common examples are certain emergency procedures. Emergency procedures by their very nature are 'unusual' and potentially life-threatening. Thus, even though a neophyte professional may need to be able to undertake such emergency procedures; opportunities to do so 'live' do not emerge; and even when they do, we would not necessarily want a learner to undertake the procedure. Learners are normally expected to practise emergency procedures in the simulation laboratory and are tested on their knowledge at regular intervals in their adult education institution. However, real-life experiences are always more dramatic and possibly frightening for learners, so having a debrief 'after the event' is a helpful way to both reassure the learner and assess their capability to take a more central role in the procedure. We will now take a detailed look at some of the assessment techniques that we described above.

Pre-practice assessment: assessment through simulation

Simulation is a widely used technique in the assessment of practical skills. Simulations are used in areas such as client consultations, basic clinical procedures and advanced operating techniques. Simulations are designed around simple or complex scenarios. It is quite common for simulations to be digitally recorded, and some may be computer-driven and involve the use of sophisticated manikins (e.g., SimMan® 3G); in other situations, actors are used as clients or are used to represent a clinical scenario. Simulations are also used to practise and to assess practical skills, interpersonal skills and communication skills in the 'classroom'.

Simulations are often used in formal assessment situations, and simulated clinical assessments are often referred to by the acronym 'OSCE' to denote 'objective structured clinical examination'. Once the preserve of summative assessments, OSCEs are being used increasingly in formative assessment.

Simulations have several useful features, the most obvious one being that they do not involve 'real' clients and thus are deemed to be safe, at least from the client's perspective. In terms of assessment, they offer the ability to establish standardised conditions; that is that during an assessment, a learner is likely to encounter the same test conditions as any other learner; also because external influences tend to be controlled, the assessment focuses on the skill of interest. Simulation also provides the opportunity to assess learners' 'on the spot' practical problem-solving skills, as it is possible in a simulation to ask 'what if questions' to test problem-solving skills and deeper understanding. When used as formal summative examination, learners often find assessment quite frightening and daunting, but in discussion, they will often be the assessments that they find most relevant.

You can appreciate that simulation is used frequently in the 'classroom' as informal assessment, but you can also use simulation in your clinical practice. You can use simulation to see how your teaching is going, for example, or to help your student get a quick feeling for their level of understanding. In Chapter 6, we illustrated a common simulation where the learner practised the technical skill of preparing for an intravenous infusion. Here, we illustrate how a mentor, Anne, assessed whether her learner, Kyle, was capable of delivering a medication by injection safely to one of her patients (see Snapshot 7.2).

Snapshot 7.2   Simulating giving an injection in practice

Kyle is on his first placement and is keen to give injections. He has practised giving them in the Skills Laboratory on the dummy but not yet on a patient. Anne, his mentor, wants to be satisfied that he knows the procedure before letting him administer a medication to a patient, so they agree that he will do a rehearsal in the treatment room, using sterile water to inject into a banana.

Kyle goes through the procedure, collecting the drug chart, washing his hands and assembling the correct equipment and a vial of sterile water. He then unwraps the equipment, retaining the sterility of the needle, breaks off the top of the vial and, using the assembled sterile needle and syringe, withdraws the fluid to the correct amount. He changes the needle and pretends to go to the patient and rehearses what he will say to the patient, screens and positions the patient, before washing his hands a second time. He then describes where he will give the injection and how he will ensure he is going to the correct site. He then goes through the procedure to administer the fluid into the banana, taking care not to cause harm. At the end of the process, Kyle explains what he will say to the patient, disposes the equipment safely and explains how he will record the medication. During the procedure Ann has been assessing his technique and giving him prompts if he seems to be faltering. When it is all completed, she invites Kyle to reflect on the experience and gives him feedback. He then repeats the procedure under her supervision, but this time with a real patient. The whole process has taken no more than 15 min but has been an valuable learning experience for both Kyle and his mentor, Anne.

Table 7.2　OSCE skill tick sheet for suturing a laceration.

Capability	Demonstrated	Not demonstrated
Appropriate introduction to patient		
Informs patient of procedure		
Confirms consent		
Opens suture pack appropriately using sterile technique		
Uses sterile gloves		
Uses needle correctly		
Uses forceps with appropriate skill		
Ties knots correctly		
Skin closure achieved		

NB: More space would be available for longer commentary. Some tick sheets may indicate degrees of performance, for example, well demonstrated/just demonstrated.

Having opportunities to practise different professional skills, such as therapeutic communication or a technical skill in a safe environment, helps learners to become familiar with the physical movements or their likely emotional response. Practice sessions, such as drawing up and injecting a solution as well as getting the feel of holding and using a syringe, not only provide a learning experience but also allow you to assess your learner's level of technical competence and so how much more practice is needed.

During simulation, an assessment of performance is normally made using direct observation. With more formal simulation-based assessments, it is normal to use a checklist to help with the assessment process. Using a checklist helps the assessor to focus on the important aspects of the skill to be observed; see Table 7.2, for an example.

Using a checklist is helpful to both the learner and the supervisor, as they both know what is required before the assessment starts. As with all assessments, it is important that everybody involved has a good idea of how they will be judged; the best way to achieve this is by doing the assessment several times and discussing the outcomes, that is, by rehearsal. This 'prior knowing' of criteria is less important in more informal assessment, but in general, professional understanding is enhanced the more we discuss what is expected. The extent to which to simulations actually are perceived as 'real' is probably the most significant criticism that is levelled at this assessment process. People often criticise OSCEs because they seek to give the assessment 'standardised' conditions. They rightly point out that such standardised and controlled conditions do not occur in reality, and as such the OSCE does not represent real life. OSCEs tend to represent practice as sets of skills that can be taught in isolation from each other. However, if we see simulation as but one tool that can be used to assess professional competence, and one that should not be used in isolation, then despite this lack of reality, it remains useful. Other critiques of simulation revolve around the cost and the nervousness that they can generate in learners. The cost of formal summative assessment using simulation can be high, particularly if actors are used. Even basic manikins can cost a significant amount, and the more sophisticated devices such as SimMan® 3G can be very expensive, although not as expensive as harming a patient! Nervousness is an emotion that most learners will feel whenever they are assessed directly or under exam conditions. Nervousness can be minimised by rehearsal, the use of relaxation techniques and, in some cases, counselling.

Pre-practice assessment: using reflection and analysis

Using simulations as discussed above are good ways of assessing someone's practical skills before they engage with practice. In addition to wanting technically skilled practitioners, we are interested in developing professionals that understand why they use a certain approach or procedure and have a deeper understanding of this element of their practice. This also applies when we ask learners to discuss and describe similar experiences that they have had in the past (see Snapshot 7.3).

Snapshot 7.3   Simulating a therapeutic interaction

Aleisha and her mentor, Sarah, work in an acute mental rehabilitation unit. Sarah feels Aleisha is ready to spend the next shift working with one of their patients who is suffering from hallucinations but wants to give Aleisha a practice run. They have a quiet 15 min, and Sarah is going to role-play the kinds of behaviour Aleisha is likely to face with Aleisha responding to the behaviour. After 5 min, Sarah de-roles and, using Socratic questions, invites Aleisha to reflect on her responses to the behaviour and what she might do differently. By the end of their 15 min session, Aleisha and Sarah are confident that she has the necessary skills to care for this patient the next day.

When using past experience and simulation to assess, we ask learners to justify and analyse their own actions and performance. The learner's elucidation of their practice thus forms the basis for an assessment of their underpinning knowledge. The degree to which emphasis will be placed on this type of assessment depends on the context; for example, it is a sign of understanding if someone can identify what they did wrong, yet we would not want this person to proceed to immediate practice for 'real' until they can demonstrate that they are safe. On the other hand, how do we manage the individual, who can perform in a simulation or describe what they did in the past yet, cannot really explain why they did what they did? This discussion again illustrates the need for assessment criteria that practitioners understand but also to know why we have them.

When analysis and elucidation of simulation are used as assessment, it is important for the facilitator to ask questions and to prompt for answers. For example, if you want someone to discuss why and how they washed their hands before touching a client, it would be a good idea to ask this specific question rather than rely on the learner to simply come up with the

---

Box 7.2   Socratic-type questions.

Questions of clarification
What do you mean by? What is your main point? How does x relate to y?
Could you put that another way? Is your basic point x or y?
Ashma, can you summarise what John has said? Could you give an example?
Could you explain that further?

Questions that probe assumptions
What are you assuming? Could we assume something else instead?
You seem to be assuming – do I understand you correctly?
Your reasoning is dependent on the fact that – Why?
What if you base your reasoning on x rather than y?

Questions about evidence
What would be an example? Why do you say that? What led you to that suggestion? How
could we find out if that is true? What would convince you otherwise? Could you explain your
reasons to us? What extra evidence do you need?

Questions about perspective
What is an alternative?
How are John's and Ashma's ideas different/similar?
Would a woman from the planet Mars have the same view?

Questions about implications
What are you implying here? When you say x are you implying y?
But if that happened, what would happen as a result?

---

reasons. Sometimes our actions become quite automatic, and we may not even mention them
when describing them to someone else. Try, for example, to describe to someone how you
might drive off in a parked car. Did you remember to describe how you got into the vehicle?
We have been using the types of questions named after the Greek philosopher, Socrates, who
believed that all knowledge could be found through questioning. These questions are useful,
both for assessment and to generate learning. Box 7.2 presents a useful collection of types of
question that you could ask and the type of 'learning' that they are probing for.

When using discussions of past experience that you have not witnessed as a basis for
assessment, you need to take care to determine if the experience being discussed was the
learner's and the reality of the experience. The implication here of course is that memory
can distort past events, and as a result we are not always honest and open with each other,
even in a professional context. It is important to remember that in a professional environment, it is very difficult to say things such as, 'No, I have never done that before', if it
is expected that you have or to say, 'I am not very good at this'. I once had a long-serving
qualified midwife say to me, 'I am not very good at helping new mothers to breastfeed'.
I was so surprised by this person's honesty and insight that I almost fell off my chair and
was impressed with her resolve to improve.

Pre-practice assessment: discussion of practice prior to practice

Discussing practice prior to engaging in it is a very good way to establish if a learner has the
sufficient background knowledge, and confidence. Simply asking someone to talk you

through a process provides considerable information. A description of practice can then be followed up with some questions that delve deeper into understanding. So, you can ask questions such as, 'Why are certain aspects of a task carried out in the way that they are or if they know of any alternatives, and if they do, what are the pros and cons of each approach?' These discussions can be extended by asking the Socratic type questions such as 'what if'-type questions? If, for example, you have asked your student how they would go about recording a client's medical history, you might ask, 'OK, what if your client has hearing difficulties, how would you obtain their medical history?' Talking your learner through a procedure or an activity is also a very useful strategy to help them learn the procedure. It can give them an opportunity to clarify any aspects they have difficulty with (see Snapshot 7.4).

Snapshot 7.4   Planning the morning's work

Matt and Sally are working together for the shift. Matt is a second-year student, and Sally has assessed him to be capable of working under her distant supervision. However, they always start their shift together, making a nursing round of their case load of patients and assessing their individual needs. Sally then gets Matt to create a plan listing his actions and the potential time they will take for the patients for whom he will be responsible over the shift. At the end of the shift, they reconvene and discuss what has been achieved and what he will be recording in his patients' case notes.

Points to ponder:

- What Socratic questions might Sally pose when discussing the morning's plan of work?
- What is Matt learning when Sally asks these questions?
- What might Sally be learning about Matt's capability from this process?

Reading through this vignette, you can probably appreciate that exercises like this can have double value. You may need to remember that when asking people to describe a particular procedure, they may not be able to recall every aspect, and you may need to prompt them. As your learners get more experienced, their routine professional practice becomes automatic, and, as so often with the most experienced professionals, they will initially struggle to give a full description of an aspect of their practice. If you are working with someone who omits many aspects, this should alert you that they may not yet have a full command of that element of their practice. It is probably helpful to try another pre-practice assessment approach.

Inevitably, if the practice you are assessing is a practical skill that must be executed faultlessly to prevent harm to your patient, discussion should not be used as the sole assessment technique. You need to use some form of simulation or rehearsal. Remember that when working with learners or supervising others, you must always be satisfied that the person to whom you are delegating the task is capable of fulfilling it safely and that you have a duty of care to your clients.

Pre-practice assessment: case studies

Using a short case study of a situation that might be experienced frequently in your clinical setting, or using a patient's case history, is a useful way of teaching as well as establishing your learner's level of knowledge and understanding. Case studies of clinical situations have advantages over discussing a learner's own past practice, as it removes the element of ownership and thus substantially increases the objectivity of the discussion. Snapshot 7.5 provides an example, and you can probably think of several that are relevant to your own clinical setting.

Snapshot 7.5   Responding to an emergency

Cathy is a third-year student on her way home from a busy shift in the local accident and emergency department. A jogger runs past her and suddenly collapses. Cathy runs up to him, checks his carotid pulse and starts cardio-pulmonary resuscitation. She shouts for help while she is doing this, in the hope that someone will hear her and come and help her.

Socratic questions:

- What do you think of Cathy's actions?
- Is there anything else she might have done before starting CPR?

A case study such as that in Snapshot 7.5 provides opportunities for discussion that can lead to learning as well as giving you a means of assessing your learner's understanding of the scenario. Using a case study of someone else's practice like this can reduce levels of anxiety, as any notion that you are interrogating and critiquing your learner's past practice is removed. A discussion of a past case can focus on discussions of why particular actions were taken, discussing alternatives and also introducing, 'what if?'-type questions. Using a patient's case histories as a basis for exploring your learner's understanding of the patient's condition and the various investigations and treatments that they have undergone provides a similar opportunity to assess knowledge as well as to teach.

Pre-practice assessment: challenge scenarios

Challenge scenarios are similar to case studies by offering a patient's incomplete story. The learner is invited to make a diagnosis or to describe what should happen next and by whom. Challenge scenarios can be a powerful tool to help you to assess aspects of your learner's understanding of a patient's clinical condition, to anticipate the possible complications or consequences of professional interventions, or lack of intervention, and ability to plan appropriate treatment or care. Like simulations, challenge scenarios put the learner in a position of leading an aspect of care delivery. Challenge scenarios, unlike case studies, will not provide the learner with the outcomes of the episode of care. They will, however, provide details of a case history and current conditions/symptoms. In some scenarios, you can also provide charts and records. Some more complex challenge scenarios can be branching, that is depending on what the learner elects to do, a separate scenario unfolds. Box 7.3 provides an example that is typical.

Challenge scenarios like this are quite complex and can be used to help a group of learners explore the signs and symptoms of Mr B and the possible treatments, or you could use it, or something similar, to help your learner articulate their understanding of the loco-motor

---

Box 7.3   Challenge scenario from an accident and emergency setting.

76-year-old Mrs Adams has been brought into her local walk-in clinic by a friend from a nearby charity shop where they both volunteer. Mrs Adams has lost some use of her left arm and some of her mobility. She is articulate and says she is feeling giddy and very tired, with a mild headache which is worsening. After taking Mrs Adams' vital signs – her blood pressure was 160/110 and her pulse rate 80 beats/minute – the admitting nurse arranges for the doctor on duty to see her as a matter of urgency. On examination, Mrs Adams has weakness in her left arm and leg with deep tendon reflex of her left ankle diminished. She has difficulty with both flexion and extension movements but no pain. She is normally fit, exercising her large dog twice a day and going swimming once a week, and she takes no medications. She says her blood pressure is normally 130/80. She asks whether she was having a stroke and whether her weakness would get worse.

Socratic questions:
What do you think is causing Mrs Adam's symptoms?
What treatments might be prescribed?
What professionals might need to be involved in treating Mrs Adams?
Does Mrs Adams need to be transferred to the local hospital after treatment?

---

system and potential problems. However, you could also assess your learner's range of knowledge and understanding by using the idea of challenge scenarios when asking simple questions such as: 'What actions would you take if an obese person has fallen onto the floor?'

As with all kinds of assessments, when designing a scenario, you need to focus on what it is that you are assessing and the criteria you will be using to assess the success or otherwise of your learner.

Point to ponder:

- Think of a common situation in your workplace that new learners find difficult to manage. Create a short scenario around the situation, along with some key questions and test it out on a learner that you are mentoring.

Pre-practice assessment: witness testimonials

Witness testimonials are, just like job references, relatively unreliable. This is because you are relying on the judgement of others, and often you do not know how that judgement has been made. When you do use witness testimonials, it is best to be able to talk to the person who is providing the testimonial; in this way you can ask questions that relate to the specific aspect of practice that you are assessing. Take care to ask precise questions, such as:

- Have you observed person x performing procedure y?
- When you observed them were they safe on all occasions?
- Did they respect the clients rights?

and so on.

It is inappropriate to rely on the person providing the witness statement to say if they have any doubts about the student's capability; you must ask this question directly. You may be inclined to be more confident if the witness testimonial is made by more senior members of staff or those of high status. Do remember, however, that you need to base your assessment on the evidence and the credence of the witness to make judgements; for example the judgement of an experienced individual that has seen your learner regularly may be more reliable than that of one who has seen your student only rarely and has little experience of what is required of the learner.

Assessments during practice: direct observation

Probably the most common method of assessment during practice is direct observation. Direct observations tend to be made either with the mentor/facilitator just as an observer or with the facilitator taking part in the delivery of care and being an observer. Essentially, the idea is that we can watch someone doing something and assess if they can do it properly. Chapters 5 and 6 have provided several examples of this. The only real difficulty here is that there needs to be general agreement of what is right. If you have participated in an the argument with a friend or a family member over how to do something such as drive the car, plan a route to a destination, sail your boat, etc., you will know that even with taken-for-granted practical activities, what constitutes doing something right can be hotly contested.

Direct observation of practice can often take part over an extended period of time or can be focussed on a particular element of practice. It is generally considered that direct observation as an assessment can lead to significant learning and development of expertise, particularly when the observations are detailed, accurate and linked to developmental feedback.

Obviously, direct observation is best used for those practical skills, which can be exposed by performance. Within this statement, there is a caution that we should not presume what a person is thinking just because they can do something correctly. Atherton (2011) cautions us against using observation of performance as a means of assessing professional skill alone, that it is important not to rely on single observations and also that there is a need for clear a understanding between all involved in the assessment about what is being assessed and the evidence required to show that a practitioner has reached the desired level of competence. Other studies remind us that a robust assessment can only really be achieved when more than one assessor is involved; this robustness is very important to achieve when dealing with summative assessments (see above). By robust, we mean that we are confident that the assessment is reliable. If two assessors get a differing result, it is an indication that the way we are assessing is not very reliable. Despite the importance of having more than one assessor, in a review of observation assessment tools used in medical education Kogan et al. (2009) found that the use of more than one observer was unusual; they also noted that observers need training to rate learners' performance reliably and to discriminate between performance levels. Using only one assessor is often attributed to cost, for assessing by direct observation is costly, probably the most expensive form of assessment, although sometimes it is the only option.

Using an assessment tool

Many assessments by direct observation rely on assessment tools. Many authors consider such tools essential. Normally, the tools consist of tick lists of skills and behaviours that must be demonstrated during the assessment. The tool covers areas that may include

Trainee's GMC Number ☐☐☐☐☐☐☐ **DOPS** Date of Assessment ☐☐☐ 20 ☐☐

Surname: Forename:

Direct Observation of Procedural Skills (DOPS) ST All levels

RC
PSYCH
ROYAL COLLEGE OF
PSYCHIATRISTS

Setting: **Gen. Hosp** ☐ **OPD** ☐ **In-patient** ☐ **Crisis/ Emergency** ☐ **CMHT** ☐

ST level of trainee: ☐

	Below standard for end of ST level			Meets standard for ST level completion	Above expected ST level standard		
	1	2	3	4	5	6	u/c
1. Understanding of indications etc.	☐	☐	☐	☐	☐	☐	☐
2. Obtains informed consent	☐	☐	☐	☐	☐	☐	☐
3. Appropriate preparation	☐	☐	☐	☐	☐	☐	☐
4. Appropriate analgesia/ sedation	☐	☐	☐	☐	☐	☐	☐
5. Technical ability	☐	☐	☐	☐	☐	☐	☐
6. Aseptic technique	☐	☐	☐	☐	☐	☐	☐
7. Seeks help where appropriate	☐	☐	☐	☐	☐	☐	☐
8. Post-procedure management	☐	☐	☐	☐	☐	☐	☐
9. Communication skills	☐	☐	☐	☐	☐	☐	☐
10. Consideration/professionalism	☐	☐	☐	☐	☐	☐	☐
11. Overall ability	☐	☐	☐	☐	☐	☐	☐

12. Based on this assessment, how would you rate the Trainee's performance at this stage of training?

	Below expectations			satisfactory	better than expected		u/c
	☐	☐	☐	☐	☐	☐	☐

Anything especially good?	Suggestions for development

Agreed action:

Assessor's position: Consultant ☐ SASG ☐ Psychologist ☐ Nurse (Band 6 or above) ☐
Other ☐ (Profession: Seniority:)
Assessor's signature......

Please print Assessor's name......

Assessor's Registration number ☐☐☐☐☐☐☐☐   Date:

Figure 7.1 DOPS form for an aspect of psychiatric practice. © Royal College of Psychiatrists 2008.

aspects specific to a particular practice such as taking and recording blood pressure, but will also include aspects of communication and social skills, which could be considered to be the more general skills of a health practitioner. Medical education in the United Kingdom has recently moved to involve many more direct assessed observations of clinical practice. These assessments are known as Direct Observations of Procedural Skills (DOPS). They were introduced in order to promote the more efficient development of clinical skills for junior doctors. You can find many examples of DOPS on the internet; Figure 7.1 shows part of one for psychiatric practice.

You can see on the form that information is requested on the clinical setting; this is important because, as we discussed above, context influences ability to perform. Indeed, the OSCE was introduced in an attempt to make the assessment of clinical skills by observation more objective. Thus, direct observation of clinical practice in the clinical setting is not always fair, because the context varies depending on the setting and the clients; this is another reason why it is important that several observations are used rather than one. Note also that the assessor can be a professional from a range of settings.

You might like to consider also the extent to which the form uses criteria to make judgements. The DOPS form makes up part of a continuous process of assessment now used in the education of doctors in the United Kingdom; you can see that the form does not refer to passing or failing, and, significantly, the identification of good practice and development needs is built into the functionality of the form.

The DOPS form does, however assume that the assessment itself is based on the observation of isolated episodes of care. For many other professions, summative assessment of professional practice is more holistic and covers the whole placement or episode of training. Nevertheless, guidance on the introduction of assessment tools for single episodes of care can have important messages for more holistic approaches. Hauer et al. (2011) suggested a number of aspects to consider when introducing tools to aid in assessment by direct observation. We have adapted some of their suggestions, which are presented in Box 7.4.

Box 7.4   Aspects to consider when undertaking an assessment via direct observation.

Define the capabilities that you are assessing, and use these to develop a tools to focus your observation. Use the development of these tools to guide the articulation of developmental benchmarks (or criteria) that characterise the expected level of performance at specific points during the period of professional education.

Make sure you know the purpose of the assessment; is it formative only, is it about checking safety, or is it mostly summative?

Don't reinvent the wheel: many validated tools for assessment of a wide range of health care practices already exist; find them and adapt them for your purpose.

Good observation skills are developed through practice and discussion; discuss with colleagues and learners, how you observe and what you look for; if you have time, try watching videos of practice together and sharing your observations. This is a great exercise for learners; as you observe, consider the feedback that you will give.

Build meaningful feedback into the direct observation process and practice providing effective feedback.

Work with your student to engage in action planning soon after each direct observation.

Encourage your learners trained to self-assess before and after the assessment episodes.

If an assessment tool is being used for summative evaluation, the assessment should be carried out at least four times before a reliable measure of competence can be achieved.

If a new tool is developed for use, try to assess its validity.

Keeping records

Direct observation of practice is different from many other forms of assessment, because more often than not, there is no permanent record of the activity upon which the assessment decision is made. An example taken from adult education institutions is learners making formal presentations as part of their programme assessment of theory. To ensure there is clear accountability for the judgements made during an assessment, it is very important to keep written records of the observations and the criteria used, as the decision of the assessment outcome may be challenged, and the records will be required to examine its legitimacy. In some circumstances, the use of video records should be considered.

Record keeping is very important; not only do records form the basis for professional development planning, but also they form a record as to why an individual was deemed competent or otherwise. In respect of professional education programmes, learners can appeal against fail decisions. The practice elements of their programmes are often the most contentious, as learners often are facing dismissal from their programme and thus jeopardising their career hopes. By contrast, the assessors are protecting the public and the good name of their profession. Often the adult education institution is forced to uphold a student's appeal because of insufficient evidence. Only too often, the record of practice experience has not been maintained (see Vignette 7.1).

Vignette 7.1   The failing student

At the end of Matt's first placement, he met with his mentor, Ann, for his final placement report. His report consisted or a number of tick boxes against the learning outcome he was expected to achieve by the end of his placement. He was shocked to find that more than half of the boxes had been ticked negatively to say he had not achieved the learning outcomes. As a result, Matt had failed his placement. The summarising comment stated: 'Matt has attended the placement punctually and regularly, and dressed appropriately. Unfortunately, he has not achieved the standard for successful completion of learning outcomes.'

Matt was seen at the university by his professional tutor, who expressed her concern at the content of the report. However, Matt was very distressed that Ann had not told him that his performance had been less than expected. He stated that he had not been given a midway report despite repeated requests and as a result had no opportunity to learn how to improve his performance.

Socratic questions: if you were to read a report like the one Matt seems to have received:

- What evidence would you expect to find that demonstrates Matt's unsatisfactory performance?
- What criteria would you expect to see Ann use to judge Matt's performance?
- When would have been the best time for Ann to warn Matt that his performance is not as high as expected?
- If Ann had communicated her concerns to Matt about his performance earlier, what else should she have done?
- If Matt appeals against the decision in his report, and it goes to a tribunal, what information would be needed by the tribunal members to support Ann's decision to fail Matt?

Whenever assessment is as a result of observation based on single incidences of care delivery or based on continuous assessment, there are common principles that need to be observed:

- observation must be consistent;
- observation must be according to a systematic plan;
- the observation plan must include criteria that both the assessor and the person being assessed understand.

When assessment is based on continuous observation of practice, these principles can be much harder to meet, as it is much less transparent as to what aspects of practice are being focussed on at what time and how it is being assessed. When using continuous assessment, you need to ensure that you discuss the process with your learner regularly and often, and that you document these meetings. As you may imagine from Vignette 7.1, regularly documenting your discussions and the agreed actions for further development not only provides evidence of your supervision but also gives your learner feedback that they can read as well as listen to. Some people are able to take more notice of feedback when it is documented rather than when it is given verbally. Even when assessment is informal, and there is no summative element, documenting conversations strengthens the learning experience and could be used to form an entry into your learner's records of professional development.

Assessment during practice: by patients, users and clients

Having service users take part in the assessment of professionals has a great deal of logic to it. After all, the users are very well placed to judge the quality of the service they have received; this is particularly the case for softer skills such as communication, professional attitudes and deportment. Working with service users in this way is also consistent with the movement to empower and give more control to the end users of services. Part of the rationale for this approach is a belief that by considering professionals as the only people capable of assessing their colleagues' and learners' fitness-to-practise limits, the capacity for a profession to change. Without an objective or personal perspective offered by an 'outsider', unsatisfactory practices that have become acceptable within the profession are perpetuated, such as the custom of putting elderly people in residential homes to bed at 6 pm.

Assessment of learners by patients, users or clients is relatively unusual, this is largely because issues relating to ethics and the processes that make users feel at ease are difficult to manage. For example, users who are asked to pass judgements on the service that they receive often perceive that a negative judgement will compromise their subsequent care.

Potential ways around these issues are to incorporate users into formative assessment processes only. In some settings, service users are invited by the learners to give them feedback after they have left the setting. This has proved a valuable tool to give learners the insight that they refused to accept from their mentor, especially when the feedback did not form part of their assessment.

When service users are involved in assessment processes, it must be made very clear to them exactly what they are being asked to do. You can achieve this by using a structured questionnaire such as the DOPS form (Figure 7.1). Obviously, some service users or their carers, by virtue of their physical or mental condition, or the context, may not be in a position to give meaningful feedback.

Assessments during practice: direct observation of group activities

Assessment of group activities using observation has obvious similarities to those described for observing individuals at practice, and the need to know what you are looking for is a paramount consideration. Assessing group activity is worth some discussion, as assessors need to be aware of both their own position and influence and the potential influence of the constituents of the group on performance.

When assessing groups, it is critical that you allow for group dynamics. Group theory tells us, for example, that groups do not perform at their maximum effectiveness until they have been formed for some time. Thus, if you are seeking to assess an individual's performance in a group, you are more likely to gain a consistent result when the functional group has formed. In some circumstances (such as emergency care), it might be expected that a group will function adequately very quickly.

Group theory also suggests that the individual personalities in a group will often dictate the roles that people assume within it and, to some extent, their performance. So, the process is complex.

If you are examining leadership skills, and a group comes together that has several natural leaders, you can expect some interesting results. Unfortunately, often the assessor has little control over group composition, and so you need to be aware of the group dynamic. You may be interested as much in the group's process as in the outcome of the processes, that is, how each individual negotiates and enacts their role within the group may be more important than whether the group achieves its goals.

Whenever you are undertaking assessment where marks or grades are being allocated, you must be clear as to whether you are giving a grade to the whole group or to the individual within the group. Group marks often cause issues, and it is a good idea to discuss these issues with the group before undertaking any assessment. Sometimes, it is helpful to discuss the criteria for each mark with the group beforehand and invite them to mark each other and the group as a whole using the criteria. Sometimes, as the assessor, you may have a significant role (consciously or not) within the group assessment.

Assessments during practice: discussion of practice as it occurs

Discussing practice with your learner is a useful form of assessment, as your conversation will help to determine the level of understanding and knowledge that underpins your learner's practice. It helps to expose what Schön (1983) terms reflection in action. Schön considered reflection in action as the process integrating experiences, feelings and theories as practice occurs. Within this concept is also the notion that through reflection, we create new understanding as an experience unfolds (see: http://www.infed.org/thinkers/et-schon.htm). If we can help our learners to reflect on their practice, it becomes a powerful assessment tool, although the ethics of doing so may be argued. However, this depends upon the types of knowledge you are assessing and whether it is for a summative or formative assessment. If your aim is to assess your learner's understanding of their actions, then getting them to think aloud and to explain their rationale while doing the task can be helpful to them as a learning experience, as well as giving you an idea of the extent and quality of their knowledge. There are, of course, some issues to be aware of, some to do with the student, others with clients.

Issues to consider when using think-aloud assessment

- Introducing discussion as an assessment tool: particularly if you are using it for formal assessment, it is reasonable that you should discuss this with your learner.
- Setting the tone for such discussions: it is probably wise to avoid starting such an assessment event with a casual informal conversation, if the purpose is a formal assessment.
- Use familiar language: new learners, in conversations with professionals, will often adopt the language and jargon of the professionals around them without fully understanding this new language; this is normal and part of the process of entering a new community of practice. Sometimes assessors are misled by apparently over-confident use of language. The flip side of this is that those who lack the confidence to use appropriate terminology also feel fearful of not being able to use it. In such circumstances, it is important to remember the interpersonal skills that you have developed as a professional, and you may need to coax their knowledge from them.
- Discussion of practice in public: this invariably involves the public, a client, patient or carer. Some people may not be happy with the professionals discussing practice as it occurs in front of them or to them. To avoid such difficulties, you can prepare the patient or carers by discussing the issue with the person concerned, to gain their understanding of the purpose and to seek their permission.
- When practice is inappropriate: you need to make a decision about what to do if your learner uses practice that is inappropriate. You will not want to embarrass your learner, yet similarly you do not want to give the impression that you allowed inappropriate practice, or to put your patient at risk if the actual practice is unsafe.

To some extent, these issues, especially concerning inappropriate or unsafe practice and discussing it in front of a client with the potential chance of embarrassment, are risks associated with this approach. If you and your learner have rehearsed the activity beforehand or you are confident that your learner is technically capable of the task, you can reduce the risk.

Points to ponder:

- Is it more likely that your learner will make a mistake if they think aloud as they conduct the procedure?
- If a mistake is made, at what point do you intervene and how will you do it?

Assessment after practice: reflective analyses or commentaries

Asking people to reflect on their actions and thinking underpinning their practice is a frequently used form of assessment. Personal reflections are often gathered in discourse or can be gathered through asking the learner to put their reflections in writing. If assessing orally, it is helpful to use the Socratic questions described in Box 7.2.

Engaging learners in reflection can be a useful assessment tool and will also aid learning, as it will generate what Schön (1983) referred to as 'reflection on practice'. It is important always to focus on what you are trying to assess, and sometimes when reflection is used as an assessment tool, it is easy to focus on the nature of the reflection rather than the learning that relates to the practice. This is not to say that reflection is not an important skill, but when we use it for assessment, we must distinguish between the process of reflection and what is being revealed through reflection. Reflection is, after all, primarily a learning tool, it is described in numerous ways, yet it lacks a clear definition.

As a definition, we suggest 'Reflection is a process of consciously considering experience in order to understand and learn from that experience'. Reflection is purposeful. It inevitably involves reliving and describing experiences, analysing why the experience occurred, how the experience occurred, evaluating your own position and role, and that of any other participants in the experience. The analysis and evaluation will almost certainly also involve questioning and reasoning about our actions. To do this successfully, there needs to be an element of critical reasoning.

There are many models of reflection, such as those of Gibbs (1988), Johns (1994) and Driscoll (2007), but it is worth reiterating that these models were designed as learning and developmental tools, not assessment tools. Therefore, if you plan to use one as an assessment tool, you need to take care. In addition, some reflective models require the reflecting person to describe and discuss their feelings and motivations for actions. This is a hard thing to achieve truthfully and openly when under the stress of an assessment and in a potentially 'hostile' environment. When using a reflective model as a assessment tool, we should not be surprised if the reflection we hear and read starts to conform to ideals of practice rather than reality.

Reflection alone can never demonstrate an individual's ability to actually perform a practical skill. It can be used effectively to help identify their underpinning knowledge and understanding, and assess their potential for future development.

Assessment after practice debrief with mentor

A debrief following a short period of practice can be very useful. The idea of debriefing started in the military. It was used to obtain information from personnel following a patrol or mission. Debriefing is also used to assess if the person can be returned to their normal duties. It is easy to see how a debrief can be extended into learning events. The debrief, as a learning event, is semi-structured, that is, the facilitator has a series of questions or steps that they follow. The questions are normally designed to be progressive such that they encourage reflection, challenge and development. In Chapters 5 and 6, we gave some examples of how you can use this technique in your everyday practice before and after delegating activities to your learner. A debrief is sometimes used following a traumatic or unexpected event. Such a debrief occurs both for the participants to come to terms with the events and for their learning. Using debrief following a traumatic event should not be used to assess your learner, although inevitably you will form a view of your learner as a result of your conversation. A debrief can also be based on your own actions that you have demonstrated to your learner. In this case, it would be for you to ask your learner to explain and discuss your actions.

Another activity, similar in some ways, to the debrief is the grand round. Grand rounds are a feature of medical education and where a practitioner presents a case study to an audience of fellow practitioners. In some cases, the patient is also involved in the presentation. Nursing rounds can have a similar function, with the learner presenting each patient to their mentor with an explanation and justification of their care plan. It is easy to see how the grand round can be adapted to be an assessment.

Self-assessment

Self-assessment is a particularly powerful technique, as it engages the learner with their own practice. It can be empowering by encouraging the learner to take control of their own learning and aims through self-assessment. Self-assessment is integral to the coaching process; when you are coaching someone, you need to persuade the learner to evaluate their own performance as honestly as possible. The coach does this by asking pertinent (Socratic) questions in relation to the goals that were previously set. The role of the coach is to help their learner to discover the truth. This aspect of the coaching process has significant messages for self-assessment, which, although very useful, can also have problems. These problems tend to fall into three broad areas: superficiality, over- or underestimating performance, and assessing the wrong thing.

Superficiality

When asked to self-assess, some learners behave a bit like teenagers: 'I was alright... not bad, etc.'; the purpose of self-assessment, however, is for learners to think deeply about their practice. One method of helping learners to do this is to ask them to discuss the evidence against which they are making their judgements. You can also ask them to suggest how they could improve and how this improvement might be measured. If assessments include standard criteria or questions, such as DOPS, then learners should have a copy so they can assess themselves against them. A potential pitfall with this approach, however, is that learners can start to simply perform to satisfy the tick sheet rather than performing with understanding.

Reliability and validity

Reliability and validity are two very important concepts in assessment. All assessments involve a measuring device; this device may not be evident, for example, when it is your own internal criteria. In formal assessments, the measuring device (standards, criteria, learning outcomes, etc.) will be more obvious as in an OSCE or a DOPS (see above). As with any measurement device (e.g., a thermometer), its effective use depends on the devices being reliable and valid.

Reliability

By reliability, we mean that the device will produce the same result every time it is used. This means that it will produce the same result regardless of when it is used or who uses it. So, for any assessment of practice, we should ask, 'Would another colleague using the same device come to very similar conclusions about the ability of the person being assessed to practise?'

Achieving reliability when the measuring device is your own internal criteria of what is expected is, on the surface, more difficult than when those criteria are explicit, and more obvious measurement tools are used. However, even when assessments such as OSCEs are used, they rely on an individual judgement; furthermore, many measurement tools, because practice is holistic and complex, fail to capture the true nature of practice. A further problem discovered is that even when explicit criteria are developed, practitioners tend to defer to more hidden and holistic criteria (Parker 2009). Parker found that even when clinical assessors of nursing students were supplied with an assessment tool, they chose to use the tool as guidance and relied on 'gut instinct'. Further investigation revealed that this 'gut instinct' focused on four professional and social behaviours: student's interest, motivation and enthusiasm; communications skills; requests for help; and teamwork.

Points to ponder:

- How likely do you think another colleague using the same assessment criteria will come to the same conclusions as you about: (1) a technical skill performance; (2) a communication; (3) attitudes and comportment?
- To what extent do you think learners from the same stage in their programme but with different clinical experiences will demonstrate exactly the same level of skill performance after the same length of time in your work setting?

Validity

If an assessment is valid, it measures exactly what it purports to measure. If you take the example of an OSCE that seeks to measure communication skills, you would need to ask whether this OSCE is really measuring communication skills and whether it is doing so in the way and context that you need it to. Does the OSCE really test communication as it is done in practice? In asking this question, you also need to consider any factors that can influence the outcome of the assessment. For OSCEs, the factor that obviously springs to mind is anxiety. It is not uncommon, for example, for experienced practitioners to fail OSCEs in competencies that their mentors will guarantee that they can demonstrate in practice well. If you think back to when you did exams, do you consider that the exam was testing what you had learnt or your ability to do exams? If it is the latter, this assessment was not valid. Unfortunately, no assessment in education is completely valid.

Validity is one of the phenomena of assessment that cause most debate (although people do not often notice that they are debating validity). When our learners consider an assessment to be unfair, it is often a good indication that the assessment in some way lacks validity.

Points to ponder:
Consider the range of assessments that you have experienced:

- Were the assessments valid? Why do you think this?
- Did you have any issues with the assessments? Were they fair? Were some assessments better than others? Why?

To improve validity, you must be clear of exactly what you are assessing, and the expectations of learners should be written down and discussed with learners being assessed. Have your assessment reviewed by your peers and learners. If possible, cross-reference your assessment with other assessments. In other words, do not rely on just one method to make your judgements. Do also revisit the areas that have been assessed to determine if your learners have retained the knowledge and understanding that you have previously assessed. 'Practice makes perfect' is not only relevant to skills but also relevant to knowledge retention.

Role of an assessment strategy

If we argue that approaches to assessment are techniques or tools, then an assessment strategy is a combination of these techniques to produce an overall view of your learner's competence and capability. Using a combination of different assessment tools increases the overall validity of your judgement. Few assessments used alone have the ability to measure the full range of a particular skill or capability (see Bjørk's Skill Assessment Tool in Chapter 6 as an example of the complexity). By combining several different assessment tools, you can gain a more rounded overview of your learner's ability, which is less tainted by problems of validity. An assessment strategy needs to build up different techniques of assessment so that the overall goal of the assessment strategy is achieved. While most assessments of practice focus on issues of the assessment of skills and capability, many educationalists now recognise that an important element of assessment is that it can drive how and what is seen as important to learn. Thus, sometimes the goals of an assessment strategy include how we want it to influence learning.

An assessment strategy should also involve evaluation of its effectiveness. Such an evaluation would ask questions such as:

- Did the assessments allow learners to demonstrate the full range of competencies associated with this activity?
- Was the assessment reliable?
- How easy was it to make judgements?
- What were the learners' views on the assessments?
- Did the assessment measure what you want to at the right level?
- How many learners do not complete/fail the assessment?
- Do you feel confident in the assessment?
- How could you make it better?

Failing learners

If you are regularly involved in formally assessing learners, then that at some point in your career you will come to the conclusion that their performance is unsatisfactory and that you need to fail them. Even if you are not involved in formal assessment, as a facilitator of learning it is likely that you will meet situations where a learner does not meet professional standards: either your professional code of conduct or standards of performance normally expected of learners at their stage in their programme. Alternatively, in your capacity as a professional practitioner, your employer may require you to make assessments on colleagues.

Failing learners is difficult, and research certainly indicates that more learners should be failed than is actually the case. Reasons giving for not failing learners include the following:

- it is time-consuming;
- it creates emotional difficulties and stress;
- mentors often feel they have failed their learner.

The emotional difficulty may stem from the close relationship between learner and mentor that is necessary to create an effective learning environment. However, even in such close relationships, it is important to have clear professional boundaries between mentor and learner in order to fulfil your duty of care towards your patients. This difficulty is compounded by the fact that mentors are often expected to integrate learners into their teams where performance is based around a series of complex relationships and relationship types. Facilitators that work with adult education institutions (AEI) are often heard to complain that they feel unsupported by the AEI when they make the decision to fail their learner.

It is of course a worrying situation for patients and the good standing of professions if people are deemed to be competent when in fact they are not. You may be aware of a colleague who you do not consider to be competent, and yet they have become a registered professional on the basis of assessments by a number of other professionals, possibly within your institution. So, failing to fail an unsatisfactory learner has serious implications not only for your patients but also for you and your colleagues and their ability to function effectively as a team.

Here are some pointers that will help you fail one of your learners, should you have to:

- failure should come as no surprise to the learner;
- if there are issues of competence, discuss these with your learner at the earliest opportunity – do not leave it until there is no time to improve;
- document your discussions;
- document an action plan that has been agreed to help your learner to improve with the time and date;
- documentation of discussions should be agreed as accurate, by both you and your learner;
- follow up any agreed actions with an evaluation of progress at the agreed date – document the findings and make a further action plan if necessary;
- if you have concerns about your learner's professional conduct (punctuality, dress, attitude, etc.) tell them immediately, and document the time and date of the conversation;

- confront any issues of competence immediately they are observed – the longer you wait, the more the undesirable practice will become established, and the harder it will be for your learner to relearn and to change;
- include your colleagues (including academic and senior management colleagues) in discussions about your learner's competence – make sure that your learner is aware that you are doing this;
- when making an assessment of capability and competence, ensure you are using criteria that are appropriate for your learner at their stage in their programme;
- if you are involved in formal education, make sure that you have documented evidence of your assessments, and if necessary attach a copy of these to the end-of-placement record;
- unless most of your learners tend to fail, it is safe to say that it is highly unlikely that a student's failure is your fault.

Remember that failing an incompetent student is your professional duty and could save lives.

Improving your assessment skills

There are a number of ways we can go about improving our assessment skills. It is important that assessors be knowledgeable of their own professional practice as well as of assessment practice. We hope that this chapter has helped you with the latter. Maintaining your professional knowledge and the assessment strategy of the programme your learners are following as well as keeping up to date with different methods of assessment is very important. A good place to look for developments in assessment strategies is the United Kingdom's Higher Education Academy's (HEA) web pages. The HEA supports the development of Higher Education practice, and its web pages (http://www.heacademy.ac.uk/) contain resources that cover the whole of the higher-education sector, including health and social care. Most of its resources are free and downloadable.

Continually questioning how and what you are assessing is a vital aspect of working as an assessor. You can ask whether the assessment tool that you are using is actually measuring what you think it is. Check out your own responses to the questions discussed in the section on validity and strategy frequently and often. Ask yourself whether your assessments give you the right type of information. Do they indicate the areas that you and your learner need to focus on in order to improve? Are your assessments failing the right people? If not, why not?

Do not be afraid to change and experiment. There is an old adage that is pertinent here: 'If we always do what we always did, we will always get what we always got!' In other words, if you are not happy with how the assessment process that you are using works, takes steps to voice your concerns in the appropriate places, and get it changed.

Do discuss assessment issues with your colleagues and learners. There is most likely some form of support group for mentors either online or in your workplace. If there is not one in your workplace, why not set one up? Having a collective understanding of what it is to be a professional in your area of work and the ways in which you assess whether your learners have the necessary qualities and knowledge gives them a better chance to do well, even if they seem to be failing initially. Assessment should be, as far as possible, a transparent process. The heart of professional development is the kinds of discussions with colleagues that generate mutual learning, debate and improvement.

Summary

Assessment is a vital aspect of a mentor's role, whether you are involved in formal or informal education. Assessment is a complex and contentious process that can generate anxiety. Having an understanding between assessors and learners of what is being assessed is critical, although rigidly defining what is being assessed is difficult. There are many methods available to help make judgements, and it is best to use a variety of methods as part of an assessment strategy that needs to be evaluated and reviewed regularly. Remember that although your learner may at first appear to be weak or to be failing, most learners want to be successful and will respond to guidance and support.

Chapter 8

Giving feedback and documenting progress

Ian Scott

Introduction

In Chapter 7, we looked at assessment, in this chapter we will look at one of the most significant outcomes of assessment which is feedback. Feedback is considered, by many, to be fundamental to learning. In a large meta-study (study of studies), Hattie (1992) (as cited by Atherton 2011) found that the most significant moderator of achievement (in learning) as measured by assessment was feedback. Without feedback, can we really know what we have learnt? Can we know whether our learning is right, whether it is appropriate and sufficient? Without feedback, we may find it difficult to locate what learning we need to do next. We derive feedback from several sources, mostly from others, but also the environment, and we give feedback to ourselves. As a facilitator, you need to understand both how to give feedback and how learners may give feedback to themselves. Understanding the process of feedback is important because feedback has the potential to make learning a positive experience, but you may know from personal experience that when it is done badly, it can be a very negative experience and a significant barrier to learning.

This chapter includes the following:

- what is feedback;
- why give feedback;
- types of feedback;
- approaches to feedback;
- receiving feedback;
- improving the feedback I give;
- documenting feedback;
- improving the effectiveness of feedback that you give.

Points to ponder:

- Consider when you last received some feedback in your professional life.
- How did it feel?
- Did you learn from the feedback?

Practice-Based Learning in Nursing, Health and Social Care: Mentorship, Facilitation and Supervision, First Edition. Ian Scott and Jenny Spouse.
© 2013 John Wiley & Sons, Ltd. Published 2013 by John Wiley & Sons, Ltd.

- What kind of experience was it?
- Was it a positive or a negative experience?
- What have you learned as a result of the feedback?
- Is there anything in the way you give feedback that you may change as a result of the experience?

Feedback: some basics from theory

Feedback is a fundamental aspect of how we, as human beings, learn things. Consider how you learn which things taste pleasant and those that do not. The feedback of the sensation of pleasurable tastes or not-so-pleasant tastes ensures that we quickly learn foods that we like and foods that we do not like.

Feedback and systems

Outside education, feedback is a term used for controlling systems. You are probably familiar, for example, with heating systems being controlled by a thermostat. In this system, the heat generator (e.g., boiler) is controlled by a thermostat. The thermostat is set at a desired temperature. The thermostat both measures the temperature and relays feedback to the boiler. When the desired temperature is reached, the thermostat sends a feedback signal back to the boiler to turn it off. Using this as an analogy for feedback in education, the person making the assessment is the thermostat; they measure how close the learner is to the standard (in this analogy, the desired temperature) and relay feedback to the learner; hopefully, the learner then responds to achieve or maintain the standard required. While this is a grossly oversimplified analogy of a deeply psycho-sociological process, it does nevertheless describe what underpins some of the thinking behind feedback. This thinking would be regarded by some, particularly the Constructivist theorists, as old-fashioned; however, if you examine your experiences of feedback, you will see how it sometimes accords with this description. Feedback, as described above, would accord with the work of a group of educationalists known as the behaviourists.

The behaviourist in particular believed in the process of associative learning. This is when learning takes place as a result of a stimulus. They saw feedback as a significant aspect of the conditioning process. The most famous of the behaviourists was the Russian Ivan Pavlov (1849–1936). Pavlov's work showed clearly that quite basic behaviours can be generated and associated, through training, in response to different types of stimuli, creating what is known as classical conditioning. Building on from Pavlov's work, the American, B.F. Skinner (1904–1990), developed the theory of operant conditioning, described as a process of generating learning that is not associated with a natural process, but is as a result of training with rewards, to operate in a particular manner (Skinner 1953). Both these behaviourist psychologists used animals in their experiments and argued that their findings have relevance for human behaviour, such as having light when you turn on a switch. In operant conditioning, changes in behaviour (learning) are seen as the result of an individual's responses to events (or stimuli) that occur in the environment. In mentoring situations, you can use practical experiences as stimuli to create learning

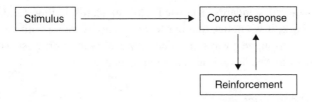

Figure 8.1   Conditioning response.

opportunities. A response is what the learner does as a result of the stimuli. In operant conditioning, when the appropriate or correct response occurs it is reinforced by the success of the action (and positive feedback perhaps).

When a particular stimulus–response pattern is reinforced, the individual (learner) becomes conditioned to respond in a particular way to the particular stimulus, and this is illustrated in Figure 8.1.

Reinforcement may be through rewards, such as positive feedback or success at the task. Alternatively, an inappropriate response may be discouraged, perhaps by failure in the task or by receiving other kinds of negative feedback. Described like this, the role of feedback is motivational, as it does not in itself convey information regarding the appropriate or desired behaviour. Skinner (1953) certainly developed to extremes his ideas around behaviourist learning. The extent to which his theories can be applied to deeper types of learning is highly debatable. However, it is also easy to see aspects of professional learning where this type of 'reinforcement feedback' is appropriate.

The role of standards

If you think back to your school days, you may recall how feedback by your teachers was used to help you learn how to read and write. Normally, you would attempt these processes, and the teacher would correct you when you went wrong (or, hopefully, praise you when you were correct). From this example, you can recognise the connection between assessment and the feedback process. First, there is an action, followed by the gathering of information about that action (in this case, from the teacher). The information is then used to make an assessment in relation to a standard; this standard may be known to all, although sometimes just to the assessor (see the discussion in Chapter 7). If the teacher then provided information concerning how your work could be improved, you would have received feedback that you could use to develop further.

It is also worth remembering that unless the required standard is made explicit, it is probable that the learner's idea of the required standard will be different from that notion held by the assessor. This means that learners will nearly always be giving themselves feedback based on their own conceptions of what is required. If you throw a ball, for instance, you know when you have thrown it incorrectly by following its trajectory, and you pretty quickly give yourself feedback, in fact, long before an instructor has suggested that it was not your best throw. As with the ball-throwing, we actually do not need to have feedback from anyone else. We know from our own internalisation of standards when our performance has not met the standard or has exceeded it. In fact, it could be argued that a considerable amount of professional learning concerns working out and understanding what are the required standards. Knowledge of standards is thus fundamental to the process of feedback; if we notice that our learner is not working with the normal standards, then we need to suggest ways in which they can try to improve so as to reach those standards. In this way, feedback is also developmental.

Feedback and constructivism

Constructivist theorists describe learning through knowledge being developed by humans making meaning from their interactions with the environment, and thus see all experience as a learning opportunity (Kegan 1982). Taking the idea that learning is a developmental activity, Mezirow and Associates (2000) argue that learning is transformational. To achieve learning, constructivists suggest that learners need to engage actively in the process of knowledge creation or meaning making before they can actually learn from their experience.

Feedback under a constructivist view of learning is more likely to be developmental when it is given rather than as a statement, but as part of a dialogue, where the learner can discuss what is being said to check their understanding. When this takes place in a feedback session, it facilitates new learning and provides opportunities for knowledge construction. Feedback in this situation is developmental and also motivational.

Constructivist theories having developed from studies of humans (rather than animals) have influenced attitudes to education and our understanding of how learning occurs. This is because it is seen as being learner-centred rather than teacher-centred. You may recognise some aspects of constructivist theories in use from your own learning experiences. Group discussions, guided study, project work and reflective practice are educational activities that have evolved as a result of constructivist theories.

Feedback in practice

From reading the previous section, you will appreciate that the main purpose of feedback in education is to provide motivation and information that helps your learner to develop. So, when you are about to give feedback, think about your intentions. If your feedback is not motivational or developmental, stop yourself, because it probably is not feedback or is not worth saying. Feedback is always intended to motivate achievement of a higher level of performance. Feedback is information from one person to another and is often referenced to a particular standard or norm. Described like this, feedback should be easy and should work every time, but in practice, sometimes it does and sometimes it does not. So, what conditions do we need for feedback to be effective?

Conditions under which feedback is effective

Intriguingly, in a review of the effectiveness of feedback, Kluger and DeNisi (1996) found that in one-third of the studies they examined, providing feedback reduced performance. This suggests that giving and receiving feedback is a complex process.

For feedback to have a positive influence, we know that learners need to be motivated both to hear and to use the feedback. This tends to mean that their previous experience of feedback needs to be positive and that learners believe that development is achievable. So, learners need to be in a mental state that is receptive to receiving feedback. Learners also need to believe that feedback comes in a way that is valid and reliable (see Chapter 7). If feedback is based on the assessment of another human, then clearly learners need to respect that other person as someone who is capable of making unprejudiced judgements in the relevant area. So, they need to believe that the judgement is fair, and any other receiving feedback for the same performance at the same level will get the same feedback. Other influences on receptivity to feedback include the complexity of the task, the expertise of the learner and their level of anxiety.

All this means is that to be effective, feedback depends on the particular situation and context in which the feedback is given. How the same feedback is given to two different learners for the same performance could have opposite effects. Directly highlighting all the errors made by a novice learner may set them back, while the same approach to an expert may spur them on.

Hattie and Timperley (2007) identified a range of different levels of feedback; the first two levels relate to the task, and the second two relate to the person. These (adapted from Stobart 2006) are described below:

- Task level: This is normally corrective feedback and concerns whether work is accurate and whether more information is needed. Simple, rather than complex, tasks benefit from this level of feedback. This level of feedback can be seen most often in behaviourist approaches to learning.
- Process level: This addresses the processes underlying tasks or relating and extending tasks. Feedback at this level may be in terms of improving error detection and cueing strategies on more complex tasks.
- Feedback about self-regulation level: This level concerns feedback about how a learner is self-regulating their own learning. Self-regulation in learning has been described as concerning, commitment, control and confidence. Hattie and Timperley (2007) described six factors associated with self-regulation that influence the overall effectiveness of feedback: 'the capability to create internal feedback and to self-assess, the willingness to invest effort into seeking and dealing with feedback information, the degree of confidence or certainty in the correctness of the response, the attributions about success or failure, and the level of proficiency at seeking help' (p. 94).
- About the learner or self level: This type of feedback gives judgements about the learner. This is using language such as 'You're a star' and 'Good to see someone has done their reading', language that can be heard in many classrooms. The problem with this type of feedback is that it does not generate learning, although in certain circumstances it could be motivational.

Feedback still not working?

Feedback, can be totally appropriate, informative, directed at the appropriate level, and focused on the task, yet still not lead to further learning.

The learner always has options about what to do with feedback. It may be negotiated, accepted and used to help move learning forward. There can be difficulties to using the feedback. For example, the emotional reaction may be overwhelming; the effort and cost of acting on the feedback may be perceived as excessive. The learner may as a result reject your feedback and start to consider reasons for not accepting the feedback such as: how their assessors are inappropriate or did not appreciate their context. Interestingly, the author whose work we cited above (Hattie 1992 cited by Atherton 2011) changed his views on feedback. He noted that actually feedback was most powerful when it was from learner to teacher, rather than the other way around:

> It was only when I discovered that feedback was most powerful when it is from the learner to the teacher that I started to understand it better. When teachers seek, or at least are open to, feedback from learners as to what learners know, what they understand, where they make errors, when they have misconceptions, when they are not engaged – then teaching and learning can be synchronised and powerful. Feedback to teachers helps make learning visible. (Hattie 2009: 173)

Hattie's conclusions reflect the constructivist thinking that learning is best when the learner is making sense of their experiences. He illustrates the importance of discussion in feedback and that it should be dialogic, rather than just based on the empty vessel concept of the teacher giving and the learner receiving. If you use reflective practice, you will recognise the similarities and benefits of encouraging your learner to reflect on their practice and to identify any strengths and weaknesses, or what they may wish to do differently.

The personal touch

Feedback does not operate in a vacuum; even task-based feedback still involves strong emotional and motivational reactions. Facilitators, for example, are often in a more powerful position than the people they are helping to learn. This can have an influence over the nature of the dialogue and therefore the way feedback is given and received, and the perception of how it is received. Feedback giving and receiving is much harder and less effective in organisations that have a hierarchical structure, where a 'blame' culture exists or where there are professional tensions and boundaries. It is easy for people to become so used to working in such an organisation that they have developed strategies to survive. Visiting learners will have not have done so and are more likely to experience difficulties. It is also worth noting that gender, age, ethnicity and general sociocultural background will influence how we give and receive feedback.

Points to ponder:

- When you receive feedback, what do you do?
- Do you act on it, file it, bin it, modify it to suit you, believe it, find excuses for it, believe only the negatives, believe only the positives, act on the negatives, but not the positives, and rejoice in it?
- Is there anyone whose feedback you value?

Responses to your feedback

In professional settings, the customary way to give informal or formal feedback is verbally. If the assessment is formal, then written feedback should follow verbal feedback. Some people are more able to take onboard feedback if it is given to them both verbally and in writing. But written feedback can feel more threatening, because it is a documented statement, and we will discuss this more later. However, you will know that there are many situations where you can give feedback to your learner, so it is good to be on your guard, looking for opportunities, deciding whether you are going to use them, and then how to use them to best effect.

Informal feedback

Informal feedback tends to be brief; it could occur for instance when observing a learner take a patient history or deliver some form of treatment, or when debriefing them from an activity. The feedback is often highly concrete such as: 'Could I show you a different way to do that?' or 'Have your thought about Z?' You could also precede a brief discussion by saying: 'Can I give you some feedback?' Inviting your learner to explain what they were hoping to achieve and to reflect on whether they met their goals is another approach to engaging your learner in constructing their own meaning from an experience and to learn from it. Informal feedback tends to be brief and take the form of 'Task level' feedback (see Hattie & Timperley 2007 above).

Formal feedback

In Chapter 7, we discussed different forms of assessment, formative, continuous, summative and end-of-placement assessment, and that you need to make time for your learner to have feedback for each of these approaches. Formal feedback tends to be pre-planned and take place over a longer period of time. It is often labelled as a 'feedback session'. Formal feedback provides an opportunity for a wider discussion. It is much more likely to focus on process and self-regulation types of feedback. Formal feedback requires dedicated time and should always be recorded in writing.

Giving feedback some general guidance

The main role of giving feedback is to help your learner to learn what they set out to learn. Hill (2007) suggests that in order to achieve this, we must bear in mind where the learner is in relation to this goal. So, this requires a preliminary assessment followed by a developmental plan. The facilitator's task is then to identify how far the learner has progressed towards their learning goal, whether they may have gone off course and what further development is required. This may appear to be a relatively simple activity, but from our earlier discussions we know that the process can go wrong. Numerous people have looked at feedback, and as a result we can suggest some general principles about what constitutes effective feedback, and some of the common pitfalls to avoid. To examine some of this work, we will start by looking at a typology of feedback and then some dos and don'ts before moving on to look at some models.

Table 8.1   Typologies of feedback.

Often regarded as better	Often regarded as inferior
Descriptive	Evaluative
Specific	General
Behaviour	Personality
Choices	Directive

Typologies of feedback

Table 8.1 illustrates several different types of feedback, each line representing an aspect of feedback and the 'polar' extremes of each aspect. In general, those on the left of the table are considered to be more beneficial than those on the right, although this is probably an over-simplification, and much will depend on the specific need of your learner and the context in which you are giving feedback.

Descriptive feedback has its focus on describing what was observed; it does not seek to make a judgement. Evaluative feedback on the other hand attempts to evaluate what was observed in relation to a particular standard. Descriptive feedback relies on the learner relating the description of practice back to their own internalised standards of how the practice should be.

Specific feedback is always related to particular instances or examples of your learner's practice. 'When you gave Mrs Jones her insulin injection, you followed the appropriate protocol' is an example of specific feedback, as opposed to 'You normally follow appropriate protocols', which would be general feedback but probably will alert your learner to ask 'Why, only probably?' Giving specific feedback allows the learner to recognise that your feedback is authentic. The more feedback is negative and generalised, the more likely your learner will become defensive and deny the feedback. Similarly, by focusing on the positive aspects of a person's behaviour, you are more likely to extinguish the negative, especially if you demonstrate the behaviours that are being sought.

As a general rule, feedback should be about observed behaviours rather than personalities. After all, you can change your behaviour, but changing your personality is far harder, and comments about personality tend to be distrusted. It is also worth remembering that more often than not, our learner's intentions are positive, even if the outcome of their behaviour does not always match their intention. Having said that, if you remember that we suggested feedback should be either developmental or motivational, at times you may want to motivate your learner by talking about the aspects of their personality that you and others value.

The last aspect of the typologies, choices/directive, refers to moving your learner forwards as a result of your feedback. How are you going to help your learner develop further? Will you 'direct' them, or are you going to make suggestions and negotiate from a range of options, or will you let your learner decide for themselves?

Suggestions for successful feedback: some dos and don'ts

Stemming from these typologies come some dos and don'ts, which support good practice in relation to feedback.

Do:

- check that your learner is ready to receive feedback;
- be clear about what you want you want to say, and make sure that what you say is likely to result in the benefit that you hope for;
- use your learner's name or the word 'you' when giving feedback avoid the use of pronouns; giving feedback using the third person is worth avoiding;
- do not use 'third person' feedback, such as Jane says, 'You are competent at giving injections'; you must own the feedback, so instead say: 'I think you are good at giving feedback';
- emphasise the positive;
- seek clarification and be willing to discuss points with learners;
- encourage self-reflection (what would have happened if…?);
- do remember that feedback is an emotional experience, for both you and the learner;
- be honest yet tactful;
- give advice and suggestions for development;
- give feedback as soon after the event as possible;
- check feedback is understood.

Don't:

- judge your learner's personality;
- comment on things they cannot change;
- be afraid to help your learner see where improvements could be made to their practice;
- fear upsetting your learner or damaging your relationship with them;
- overload;
- be over-critical.

Models for giving feedback

Over the years, some models of giving feedback have been developed. Relatively few have been rigorously tested as to their efficacy, and comparative studies are also not easy to find. To some extent, the model you choose to use needs to relate to your way of thinking and your own values but also, and as importantly, the context in which you are working. Do you give feedback to learners in the same way as you might to a colleague who is also a qualified professional or to a colleague who is an assistant? In the next section, we will look at a few of these models.

The sandwich model

The sandwich model of feedback involves delivering a critical message sandwich between two parts of positive feedback. Snapshot 8.1 illustrates a possible dialogue (abridged).

Snapshot 8.1   Paul's case conference

Paul has been running his first client case conference attended by the client and her relatives as well as the whole range of health and social care professionals. After the conference, Paul and his mentor go to the canteen for a welcome cup of tea. Paul's mentor includes feedback like this:

Mentor: 'Paul, that was a positive client review. You managed the inputs and ensured that the meeting finished with a plan. You managed to get all the right people to the meeting. I noticed your use of humour and how you used it to make people feel at ease.'

Negative: 'Do you think you managed to give the client a voice? Could you think of ways to draw the client in more? Also, do you think Mrs Andreas spoke too much? She is the consultant, but the whole team needs to believe in the way forward.'

Positive: 'Your awareness of yourself and how you can influence conference reviews is growing. You have a clear focus on your goals, and I can see how you are striving to achieve them. Well done.'

Points to ponder:
Reading through this dialogue, how would you feel about receiving feedback in this way?
Would you focus on the positive element, the negative or both?
Would this type of feedback influence you?
Would you be wondering when the negative feedback is coming?

Notice how, in Snapshot 8.1, while the model for giving feedback is important, the actual feedback remains the most significant element; after all, the feedback could have been:

- positive: 'Paul, you handled that meeting really well';
- negative: 'Pity you didn't let the client speak much';
- positive: 'Never mind, you are getting better'.

While very commonly cited, this model does have its detractors. It is easy to see in both examples above that the approach leaves little room for dialogue. Perhaps more importantly, the model has been criticised as leaving the receiver ambivalent and not quite sure how to take both the positive and negatives. Or perhaps the learner leaves the conversation, only focusing on the positive or only hearing the negative.

Some commentators also argue that it is a method designed more for the giver than for the receiver (makes it easier to deliver negative feedback) and can be patronising to the receiver. Furthermore, the approach implicitly places significant value on the negative and corrective aspects of feedback rather than the developmental aspects.

Models that promote dialogue

Some models of feedback have been designed that systematically incorporate dialogue into the feedback process; these are often, although not exclusively, promoted to educators of medics.

Pendleton's rules

Pendleton's rules (Pendleton et al. 1984) form a model of feedback that is useful when the occasion for feedback is formal. The model promotes dialogue and has a distinct focus on positive aspects of performance and development. The Pendleton's rules approach represented an attempt to remove some of the destructive critique that medics often thought they received during clinical learning experiences. Pendleton's rules for effective feedback are as follows:

1   Check the learner wants, and is ready for, feedback.
2   Let the learner give comments/background to the material/action that is being assessed.
3   The learner states what was done well.
4   The observer(s) state(s) what was done well.
5   The learner states what could be improved.
6   The observer(s) state(s) how it could be improved.
7   An action plan for improvement is made.

As you can see, Pendleton's Rules suggest an approach that may look very formal. It does allow for dialogue and allows for recognition of what was achieved. It looks at how things can be developed and includes an action plan. The drawback of the model is that its structure is rigid and that stage 7 does not seem to let the learner take any control. In addition, it is considered by many users to be overprotective and constrains constructive criticism. Nevertheless, a structured approach such as Pendleton's rules does mean that both the learner and mentor have a built in role in the feedback process, and active and reflective learning is promoted. Another critique of Pendleton's rule is that it is too far from reality and that for some learners, there may be very little that was done well. In response to these criticisms, other writers have built on this structured approach.

Silverman's approach

Silverman's approach (Silverman et al. 1996) is structured yet clearly puts the learner at the centre; see Snapshot 8.2.

This Snapshot of the conversation between Patience and Cathy is very brief but illustrates a developing relationship between the two of them. It also illustrates some of the points that Silverman argues lead to more successful feedback. He identified six stages:

The stages of Silverman's model (slightly adapted) are:

1   Establish the learner's agenda.
2   Learner discusses the issues (problems) encountered during an event.
3   Learner reflects on the learning outcomes that need to be achieved.
4   Facilitator asks the learner to identify the help they would like.
5   Facilitator asks the learner how they could engage with these issues.
6   Learner is encouraged to look for solutions to the issues with the facilitator.

Silverman's model is based on working in an Action Learning group and so assumes that the learner will be supported by the group members and the facilitator. You can probably recognise how you can use the same processes with your learners on their own. Silverman's model is much more facilitative and aligned with a constructivist view of learning.

Snapshot 8.2   Cathy's feedback session with Patience

Patience and Cathy are sitting in a quiet office, where they know they will not be disturbed (the sign is up on the door), and their conversation goes like this:

Patience: Well Cathy this is the end of your first week working here. How are you feeling about being here?

Cathy: It is very different from the last placement, and I still feel apprehensive about being on my own with the clients in case I do something wrong. But it has been good to shadow you and my other mentor, and that is helping me to understand what I need to be doing.

Patience: Yes, it is probably very different from your last placement, so it will take time to settle in. However, we are pleased with your progress, as learners often take longer than you have to adjust. I see that you have a copy of our education programme, and I am interested to know what you think of it and if there is something you would particularly like to learn about over the next three weeks.

The conversation continues with a discussion of what Cathy would like to achieve. Once Patience and Cathy have agreed a plan, who will help Cathy and the dates for review, the information is recorded in Cathy's learning passport and signed by both of them.

Table 8.2   Descriptive feedback.

Approach A	Approach B
I think your communication skills are wonderful, a perfect start	At the beginning, you gave her your full attention and never lost eye contact – your facial expression registered your interest in what she was saying

Descriptive models

Descriptive models of feedback are based on implicitly encouraging reflection; like Silverman's model, they are non-judgemental. Using the descriptive approach, however, the mentor focuses their feedback on describing what they saw and any potential implications. The mentor does not judge if what was observed was correct, incorrect good or bad. The mentor leaves this judgement to the learner.

Point to ponder:

Comparing the comments in Table 8.2, which would you like to receive as feedback? Which is more useful? Why?

Note how Approach B, helps to remove emotion but does rely on the learner to judge whether or not the observed performance/learning is correct. Some mentors do not like this 'removal of emotion', but in the long term such an approach could help the development of a professional learning relationship. Another form of this approach is known as PI or Point Illustration. In this technique, a point is made that is then illustrated by example. This technique again tends to give non judgemental/descriptive feedback that is example-driven. Another similar technique is PEE or Point Explanation Example. This is really an extension of the PI system and is illustrated below:

Point: When you give an opinion, it is important to substantiate it with some evidence.

Explanation: Providing evidence helps your learner to see that your opinion is based on logical thoughtful process and helps them to understand how your opinion came into being.

Example: For example, 'When explaining the advantages of vaccination to a parent if you show some of the risk statistics, they may be more likely to heed your advice'.

You as the deliverer of feedback

It is clear that feedback giving is a process that depends for at least part of its success on the relationship between the feedback giver and the receiver, and that the nature of the feedback itself may be influenced by the disposition of the feedback giver. Do you, for example, have a burning desire to tell someone how it *should* be done, or are you happy to help them find out for themselves?

At times, it will be appropriate to use either one of these extremes, but you will probably find that you are naturally disposed towards one of them. When you use an approach that you are not naturally disposed towards, you will no doubt feel uncomfortable and challenged. Being aware of your preferred style will help you to accommodate other approaches.

Points to ponder:

- Think of a time when you last gave someone feedback (not necessarily a professional situation). What was the situation?
- What approach did you take?
- How would you describe your style?

When we give feedback, we can fall into a range of categories, each with their own benefits and potential pitfalls. A version of these 'categories' is shown in Figure 8.2. One of the axes, the vertical, is represented as an extreme between 'telling' the learner what was right and what was wrong, and what they should do, and the other extreme of 'laissez

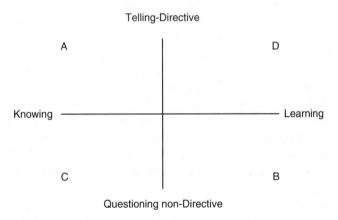

Figure 8.2   Dimensions of giving feedback.

faire', whereby the learner is left to make their own evaluation and come to their decision alone. In the middle is probably a facilitative approach where the feedback is undertaken in an environment that creates a questioning approach. The horizontal axis represents the extreme between the mentor who presents themself as an expert and the mentor who presents themself as a co-learner alongside their learner.

When combining these two axes, we can see that there are potentially four extreme types of approach or disposition, represented by the letters A to D. The quartile A is represented by mentors that view themselves as more expert than their mentees; they are happiest telling their mentees about their practice and directing them on how they should improve. Type B is the opposite; their approach is to ask their mentee questions about their practice and ask their mentee to describe their practice. They do not believe they have the answers and will seldom give an opinion. If a learner asks 'How do you think I did?', their mentor is most likely to say 'How do you think you did?' Type C mentors believe that they are more expert than their mentees but that their mentee should not automatically be told directly the best way to do something. Type C mentees can become frustrated when their mentees do not do it their way. A type D mentor would be quite unusual, as they would both want to tell the learner what was wrong and what to do but also conceive themselves as a co-learner with their mentee. Obviously positions A, B, C and D are extremes.

Points to ponder:

Using your example from your answers to the last 'Point to Ponder':

- Where would you honestly put yourself on the axis?
- Do you feel you might be able to consciously adapt your approach?

Preparing to give formal feedback

If you are going to give formal feedback to your learner, you probably have known when you need to give it and so will have time to prepare for the occasion. Used wisely, this time can help make the session go really well.

First, you need to think about where you are going to give the feedback. Normally, it should be done in a quiet and private place, free from interrruptions. You could, however, use a more public location if you are giving positive feedback, and you want to enhance an individual's self-esteem or standing with a group. Of course, such a tactic needs to be used with caution; after all, you would not want to inadvertently de-motivate another member of your team or unduly embarrass your learner. That said, most of us enjoy a bit of public acknowledgement when things are going well.

Prevent disturbance when giving feedback. If you plan ahead, and your colleagues know that it is important not to disturb you, you are less likely to be interrupted. If you are disturbed, unless it is very important, deal with the disturbance without stopping your feedback session, this will show your learner that the feedback session is important to you. Being disturbed often means losing the quality of the situation and disrupts concentration.

Prepare your learner: check that your learner knows what the session is for, how long it will last and that they are happy for the session to take place. Make sure your learner knows whether you expect them to have made any specific preparations for the session. It is also helpful to let your learner know which model of feedback you will be using. Make sure you have your notes of any observations that you or others have made, and remember to bring any necessary paperwork.

If the aim of the feedback session is to plan further development activities, make sure your learner is aware of this and that they can come prepared. During the session, it is a good idea to write down these development activities, preferably with dates by which they should be accomplished and who (if necessary) will be facilitating the activities. Writing down proposed activities and the associated learning not only provides the basis for future planning and perhaps feedback activity but also provides a sense of commitment.

Feedforward

Feedforward is becoming a popular term associated with giving feedback. The idea is to remind feedback providers that they need to work with their learner to find ways in which they (the learner) can improve. The question is no longer just 'How well did I do?' but 'What can I do to get better?'

Strategies for improvement are covered elsewhere in the other chapters, but it is important to remember that feedback is part of a package, and if we are prepared to give feedback, we must also be prepared to give constructive ideas for development or help the learner to form their own development plans. This latter point is relevant because where plans are evolved by the learner, they are more likely to be owned by the learner, the learner is more likely to feel empowered, and they are more likely to enact their plans.

Documents

If you are involved in mentoring and in assessment of your learner, it is good practice to keep records of your activities, in the same way that you keep records of your other professional activities. In formal assessments, it is almost certain that you will be asked to provide documentary evidence of your findings and the feedback that you provided. These documents are used to decide your learner's future progress towards professional qualifications or employment. In the first instance, they go to the Adult Education Institution (AEI) and the learner's professional tutor. If your learner's progress is unsatisfactory, your feedback document will probably go before an assessment panel for consideration and action. It might be necessary for your records then to be considered by an external examiner, and possibly a higher committee in the AEI, and subsequently a court of law. When these feedback records are the same documents that are used for assessments, they are used to judge whether the learner is suitable to join their profession, and so they are extremely important. It is very likely that future references are also based on the comments in these documents. Such documents may also be used as the basis for development plans, and subsequent assessments and feedback may be based on this plans.

If you envisage documentation as an opportunity to think deeply about the feedback you are giving and your assessment decision, it becomes less of a chore. Committing our thoughts to writing helps to clarify thinking and help in formulating meaningful development plans.

If you make notes during the feedback process, you should keep them in a secure location. Documentation, if required as a record of a meeting, should be completed as soon as possible either as a joint activity between the participants or immediately after the meeting. The record of the meeting should be agreed and signed by all the people present at the meeting. If agreement is not possible, it is good practice for the parties in disagreement to complete their own records, and for these records to be seen and signed as acknowledgement by each party. It is not unknown for people to remember events differently, especially when there is a high level of anxiety involved (in either party). Where feedback is formal and potentially significant to your learner's career and life, it is essential that records are kept.

Points to ponder:

- Consider one of the learners who is on placement in your setting. If you go to look at their records, is there any documented information about the standard of their performance or their attitudes?
- What information has been documented about their last (formal or informal) assessment of their performance?
- Is there an action plan to help them meet their goals and to remedy any weaknesses?
- Is there a follow-up date for reassessment of their progress?

Professional implications of documented records

The quality of records of placement assessments is a cause of frustration between providers of professional learning (AEIs) and placement providers (mentors, practitioners), especially when a failed learner is involved. AEIs and professional organisations have become concerned that a significant number of learners pass practice placements when they should be failed. The repost from clinical practitioners is often that they are not supported when they want to fail learners. The reason for the perceived lack of support from the AEI is the poor quality of evidence supplied by the practitioners. Like many providers of services, decisions whether to pass or fail a learner and whether the learner can continue or be dismissed from their programme rely on convincing evidence that the learner has failed when given every opportunity to improve. The decision by an AEI to fail a learner is likely to be challenged by the learner supported by their union representative, and they can go onto a legal challenge if there is insufficient robust evidence.

Challenges to a decision

Normally, a challenge is based on the processes rather than the outcome of the assessment. Learners cannot argue that the assessment decision was wrong, but they are able to challenge the decision if the required processes were not actually followed, or if there is no (documented) evidence that processes were followed appropriately. Most successful challenges are achieved because there was no (documented) evidence that the 'failing learner' was made aware of their shortcomings and given time to improve. Evidence of being given time to improve includes an action plan following assessment, and a subsequent assessment after a reasonable lapse of time to assess progress and a subsequent action plan. Documentary evidence is a vital part of the evidence, and normally learners are given the benefit of the doubt and opportunities to improve. A learner who is failing consistently does take up a huge amount of everyone's time. But if it leads to public protection, it must be time spent well.

Inevitably, with public concern about professional practice and regular incidents or people coming to harm as a result of malpractice, the professional bodies are putting into place strategies intended to hold professionals to account over their decisions about a learner's fitness to practise and to qualify.

Improving your feedback

Most of us have had some experience of giving feedback or receiving it. If you want to improve your feedback, try thinking back, using what you have learned in this chapter, and consider what you could have done to improve that feedback. Consider, particularly, its effectiveness. The most important measure of the successful feedback is probably whether it leads to positive change in the receiver or if it discourages development. Another way to improve your feedback is to evaluate its effectiveness. To do this, you may want to ask yourself the following questions about your feedback (or feedback you received):

- It was effective because. . . .?
- Why did the behaviour change as a result of the feedback?
- The behaviour change was what I expected – why?
- What did I feel while giving/receiving feedback? Why?
- What was the other person feeling while receiving/giving feedback?
- Will any documents generated be used and useful in the future? Why?
- How might I change the feedback and the way it was given to make it less effective?
- How might I change the feedback and the way it was given to make it more effective?

Of all these questions, the first is probably the most important, so if your time is limited this is the one that is most useful. Of course, measuring effectiveness is not necessarily easy, but the focus should be on observed change. Notice that we have not suggested that you ask your learner. In general, asking your learner is an excellent way of obtaining feedback, but such feedback is less useful in situations where there is a one-to-one learner/mentor relationship, as the learner may feel that their feedback will hinder the quality of their relationship with their mentor.

Exposing your feedback to others is another effective way of improving your feedback. Oddly, such practice is relatively unusual. This is probably because giving feedback is a largely private process. Having someone observe your feedback can be a very powerful way of obtaining feedback on the way you do it. You will need to think carefully about whom to invite to observe your practice. As we have stressed earlier, the conditions under which feedback is given influence how well the receiver will benefit from the process.

The same applies to you, so your chosen observer will need to be someone you respect and who is prepared to take the risk of giving you an honest, professional evaluation. If you do not feel up to this, you could ask someone to review your written feedback, or you may like to try making an audio or visual recording of a feedback session, after gaining your learner's consent. You can watch the recording and make reflective notes as you go through it. As with any activity, watching how others do something is a helpful way to learn.

If you choose to receive feedback on any aspect of your work:

- try to focus on what you hear, and focus on the elements that are constructive (not all people giving feedback will be good at it);
- try not to think about a response or justification but think about what you are gaining from the feedback;
- do remember to ask for suggestions and offer to reciprocate by observing the person that observed you.

Practising giving feedback can lead to improvement, particularly when working through some of the models described above. When practising feedback, use real situations that are low stakes. You can think of suitable situations when you are working with secure and accomplished colleagues. Alternatively, there may be situations that are more domestic than clinical when you can practice with a partner or family member at home.

When you are practising to give feedback, remember:

- plan your approach;
- be alert to your use of language;
- consider the effectiveness of your feedback;
- don't forget that even in low-stakes situations, people still have emotions.

Summary

Feedback helps everyone to monitor their progress and to make sense of what we are learning. Feedback is part of our everyday lives. In your role of mentor, your aim is to facilitate another person's growth and development. You need to use feedback as a way that allows their growth to help them to achieve their goals. Given that feedback is so fundamental to effective learning, choosing the appropriate approach to giving feedback is important. There are various methods to giving feedback, and as a mentor it is helpful to discuss with your learner how best to give it. Although the way most of us give feedback is linked to our personality, being sensitive to our learner's needs and to adapt appropriately increases the likelihood of success. The very act of discussing the issue with your learner will create a stronger bond between you that enables honesty and openness.

Chapter 9

Inquiring into personal professional practice

Ian Scott

Introduction

This chapter is based on the notion of 'action inquiry', and using this concept, we explore approaches to inquiry such as: reflection, using empirical data, action learning sets and AI. The chapter focuses on exploring action inquiry in relation to developing your practice as a facilitator of learning, but also as a process that you can use to help your learners develop. Action inquiry is a valuable tool to improving workplaces and organisations. We will explain the difference between action inquiry and action research.

This chapter includes the following:

- the concept of action inquiry;
- how to investigate your own practice;
- the art of reflection;
- the role of empirical evidence;
- type of evidence;
- levels of evaluation;
- approaches to group inquiry.

Inquiring into personal professional practice

This chapter explores ways in which you can investigate and inquire into your own practice. You may want to do this for two reasons: you are intrinsically interested in the way you undertake your professional role; and you wish to improve and develop. Both these reasons are quite basic human desires, as many of us are driven to improve both ourselves and the world we see around us. Therefore, the act of exploring our practice should be commonplace.

In this chapter, we shall explore how to use action inquiry as an approach to personal and group development. This approach uses the view that our own actions are worthy of personal research. The more common approach to inquiring into personal professional development is to engage in reflective practice. Despite reflection being a very natural

Practice-Based Learning in Nursing, Health and Social Care: Mentorship, Facilitation and Supervision,
First Edition. Ian Scott and Jenny Spouse.
© 2013 John Wiley & Sons, Ltd. Published 2013 by John Wiley & Sons, Ltd.

process, in our experience we have found that the mere mention of the term 'reflection' tends to put people off. We see reflection as being one of the tools of action inquiry, but not the only one. We also recognise that many people do not see themselves as 'natural reflectors' particularly in a formal way.

What is action inquiry?

First, action inquiry perceives every action as both a process of inquiry and worthy of inquiry. When we act, we are always subconsciously asking the question, 'What if', or even, 'Will the same happen?' In effect, every action is an experiment. Second, action inquiry sees each inquiry as an action in itself (Torbert 2010). Perhaps more simply put, action inquiry is the active attempt to learn while performing actions, with the intent that this act of learning will enhance the actions.

Action inquiry falls under the banner of research processes known as 'action research' (sensu Lewin 1948). Action research has a focus on researching change, where the researcher is both the person giving rise to the change and the person undertaking the research. The purpose of action research is simultaneously to generate change and to carry and evaluate that change. A simple diagram of the action research process is shown in Figure 9.1.

In Figure 9.1, the 'Observe' box is synonymous with data gathering; 'Considering' is the process of analysing, and thinking about and interpreting the meaning of these data. 'Act' is to put into action those plans, which will lead you back to making observations of those actions. 'Planning' is the formulation of any action that you may take to make a change. Note how this action research cycle is a spiral rather than a circle.

In action research, it is normally a process or way of working that is the subject of the change. In action inquiry, it is more often a person, and action inquiry may take place

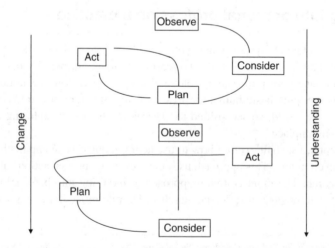

Figure 9.1 Diagrammatic representation of the action research spiral.

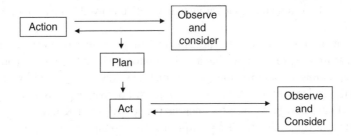

Figure 9.2   Diagrammatic representation of action inquiry.

without a simultaneous change. Indeed, in action inquiry, the purpose may be to increase understanding of personal everyday practice and that there is no explicit link between acting and observing (Figure 9.2). Action inquiry is as much about understanding everyday practice as it is about changing it.

Within action inquiry, many approaches to inquiry are legitimate, and everyday action can be as important to consider as the exception questions. Questions such as 'Why do we do it like that?' and 'Why did that happen?' are both equally relevant. Action inquiry is also distinguished by the fact that it is often collaborative and can occur at different levels with an organisation.

If all members of an organisation, or at least units within an organisation, are engaged in action inquiry, the formation of effective communities of practice should be much more effective.

Action inquiry can thus be person-centred, focused on your own personal practice; group-based, where two or more people inquire into a phenomenon of mutual concern; and finally organisational, where a group looks at effecting change across the whole organisation. In this chapter, we will focus on the first two of these, but we will also touch on the third.

Using action inquiry in everyday practice

When you are providing mentorship and facilitating another person's learning, there are several aspects of your role that you could investigate. For example, you could look at your own function and success as a facilitator; you could look at such things as how, within a group of mentors, you create an effective learning environment or at an organisational level at how your workplace welcomes new learners.

Action inquirers will want to pose questions about their day-to-day practice. They need to use the question 'Why?'. Your aim in undertaking Action inquiry is to increase the amount of evidence that is known about the phenomena of interest. It includes trying to understand the philosophical background behind particular practices. Why, for instance, do we value diversity, and where does this valuing of diversity come from? In asking these kinds of questions, action inquiry can lead to the development of more choices, options and greater understanding of alternative ways of thinking and of practising. Action inquirers will often seek to examine and explore the positions that they hold.

Action inquiry also often helps in learning to live with unsolved issues, contradictions and compromise.

We are not proposing here that vast amounts of your time be given over to action inquiry. What we are proposing is that as a facilitator, it should become a natural part of your practice, almost a sub-conscious part. Sometimes, however, you will want to engage more formally and systematically in action inquiry. For instance, having a high success rate as a facilitator may be a cause for undertaking some formal action inquiry to find out what it is that you are doing that is so unique and successful.

Role of reflection in action inquiry

What is reflection?

Reflection is the perfectly natural human act of looking back at past events that were either observed or experienced directly and trying to make sense of them. In many models of reflection, there also exists a purposeful intention to use reflection as a tool to aid improvement and development. Action inquiry, with its focus on 'understanding', does not necessarily lead to an 'action'. Unfortunately, many practitioners seem to wince at the word 'reflection'. We suspect that for many practitioners, this is because it has been linked to assessment of practice. As professionals, we all need to analyse and explore our own practice, and you will appreciate from reading Chapter 8 that reflection is one way of self-development and so to achieving this. Where academic programmes have used reflection as an assessment, they have found that learners tend to write about their practice in a way they believe their assessors want, rather than searching for the 'true' nature of their practice. Another misconception of using reflection as an assessment tool has been the inclusion of personal thoughts and feelings, thus exposing the writer to inappropriate criticism. Care also needs to be taken that individual self-evaluation seldom reflects the evaluation of others; thus, evaluation of practice through reflection needs to be conducted sensitively.

Models of reflection

Gibbs's reflective cycle is probably one of the most well-known reflective models (Figure 9.3). This reflective cycle has several stages: description, feelings, evaluation, analysis, conclusions (general), conclusions (specific) and action plan. In some ways, it should be seen as a spiral rather than a cycle, for the actions will lead to yet more observations, and so the process will continue. The stages of the Gibbs reflective cycle can be seen in most reflective models, so we will describe these stages before briefly discussing a few of the more common models.

Many people struggle to find something to write about believing should it be a big 'Event'. However, action inquiry encourages us to look at everyday events from our life, so perhaps even if the event was not particularly good or bad, perhaps it was ordinary. In fact, we suggest that ordinary is actually well worth celebrating and investigating, simply because it is something you do everyday!

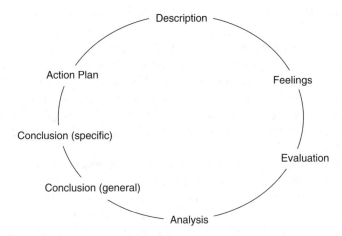

Figure 9.3   Gibbs's reflective cycle. (Reproduced with the kind permission of the Oxford Centre for Staff and Learning Development, Oxford Brookes University, UK)

Describing your experiences

As with most models, it starts with a description of events, the idea being that the description should be as objective as possible. Of course, this is seldom possible: first, because those experiencing the same event will notice different things; and second, we all have selective and porous memories. If you are intending to use reflection to develop your practice, it is best to keep a record of suitable events as soon as possible after they happen. This does, however, beg the question: what is a worthy event? The action inquiry approach recognises every day actions as worthy of exploration; thus normal everyday professional activities, such as feeding a patient or encouraging daily exercises, need to be regarded as significant. Using the Gibbs reflective cycle, it is best not to make any judgements or to evaluate your actions while you are in this description phase. Your description should be as full as possible. For example, saying that, 'Your *client entered the room and you invited her to sit down*', is qualitatively different from saying, 'Your client, who was a 25-year-old female, looking gaunt and anxious, entered the room, and you invited her to sit down at a chair at right angles to your desk'.

The level of description and what is described are important, because this description is analogous to the 'data' in a traditional, qualitative research study. Your description will influence what you will learn. This is because your description is a record of what you, the observer, thought was worthy to be noted and so, by default, what was not worthy. So, your own learning will be either restricted or enhanced by your own 'lens,' just as with a photograph whereby you only record what you point the lens at. You may feel that some people are better at describing, but with practice it is possible to improve what you think is worth describing.

There are a number of approaches that you can take to improve your observation skills. For example, after you have had an 'experience', try noting five points about it, then try to add five more, then another five. Each point does not need to seem significant, but often you will find that an insignificant point becomes much more pertinent, once you have thought about it.

You are probably good at observing other people and noticing nuances of their appearance and their behaviour, but are you as good at using your internal eye and monitoring your own actions and speech? You may find it helpful to practise recording everyday activities, such as preparing a meal, or your interactions with the checkout assistant at your local shop and so on. Another approach to improving your observation and recording skills is to visit a 'place of interest' such as a local museum, art gallery or park, and spend time recording the individual features of any objects that catch your eye. Try spending 15 min with one object noting down as much as you can; even better, try going with a friend or your family and compare notes.

If you go to meetings as part of your work or home life, practice making a note of what you consider to be the important points, and then compare your notes with the minutes of the meeting. This technique can also help increase your self-confidence and improve your performance at meetings. Another significant aspect of observing is to have some knowledge about the activity you are observing; the more you know about, the more you will see. For example, if you know a fair bit about a particular sport, when you watch it you tend to notice more than the uninitiated. Some people are better at learning and remembering things using diagrams, cartoons, drawings or audio-recordings, so you may find using one of these different ways to record events more helpful as a prompt to recall different aspects of an experience.

Identifying your feelings

Gibbs's model explicitly mentions feelings. This acknowledges the importance of feelings that influence all experiences either indirectly or directly, and there will always be an emotional response. In most interpretations of the Gibbs cycle, you are simply asked to describe what you were feeling; of course, post-event, this may be difficult. Educationalist, David Boud (Boud et al. 1985), has also written extensively about reflection, and his model of reflection also includes a section: 'Attend to feelings'. He recognises that feelings are something to be recognised and acknowledged but also need servicing. They need to be recognised so that they do not interfere too much with the 'making sense part' of reflection. Boud and his colleagues argue that recognition of feelings is an important part of the event. Sometimes, if you are reflecting on a particularly difficult event, you will not be able to move on to the 'making sense stages' until you recognise and acknowledge your feelings at the time, and perhaps subsequently.

Socratic questions you could ask yourself are:

- 'How were you feeling at the start of the experience?'
- 'How did those feelings develop during the experience?'
- 'Were your feelings influenced by other people around you?'
- 'If your colleagues were involved, how do you think your colleagues were feeling?'
- 'If there was a client/patient, how might they have been feeling?'
- 'Would your feelings have been different if you were with a different group of people?'
- 'As the event came to an end, how would you describe your emotional state?'
- 'What do you feel about the event now?'

You could also introduce 'why'-type questions, for example, 'Why were you feeling the way that you were and what factors were influencing you?' Most of us concentrate on the negative feelings, so it is important to remember the positive ones as well. Using reflective practice can be challenging and, for some people, stressful as past memories come surging to the surface. If you find that you are feeling overwhelmed or distracted by these memories, it is well worth seeking help from a friend or a professional. Some people consider that emotion is the most significant trigger of refection (Johns 2000), so perhaps we should consider redrawing Gibbs's reflective cycle with 'Feelings' as the starting point.

Evaluation

To us, this stage of the cycle seems slightly poorly named, in that normally we would expect to see evaluation coming after analysis. We describe analysis as 'the art of deconstructing and taking apart a phenomenon' (as in chemical analysis). Here, however, the Gibbs model asks you to make a relatively 'quick and dirty' judgement of what went well and what did not; what was good about the experience and what was not. This tends to suggest that experiences can always be judged in this way, which of course is not often the case. The requirement to make a judgement so early in your reflective process is perhaps counter-intuitive when using a deeply analytical process like this. It is quite common for us to judge our own actions immediately, or even during the event. It could be argued that following the Gibbs cycle and putting those judgements into writing could inhibit attempts to generate understanding. In terms of action inquiry, you may actually miss out this stage, even though you could learn a great deal by following it through.

Analysis

A simple definition of analysis is that it is the process of breaking down a complex issue (or substance) into smaller parts so that we gain a better understanding of the whole. In the context of reflection, it normally means seeking causes and explanations for the events that are being studied. These explanations may be drawn from previous experiences, talking to others or looking at the literature. Gibbs's own words are useful (Gibbs 1988) here; he offers some questions for going through the process at this stage:

- 'What sense can you make of the situation? Bring in ideas from outside the experience to help you.'
- 'What was really going on?'
- 'Were different people's experiences similar or different in important ways?'

Notice how Gibbs's questions lend themselves to providing discursive responses. Other useful questions are Rudyard Kipling's four other friends: 'How?', 'What?', When?' and 'Where', for example:

- 'When did this take place?'
- 'What preparations did I make?'
- 'Why did I use this technique?'

- 'How effective was this approach?'
- 'How did the client respond?'
- 'What was different with this situation as compared with yesterday?'

If you have read Chapter 7, you might notice that these are similar to the Socratic questions that we described. They are also useful for analysing descriptions in reflection. The Socratic Method is based on a method of analysis devised by the classical Greek philosopher, Socrates (Scott 2004). Socrates believed that by continuing to ask these kinds of questions, he would eventually discover the ultimate truth. Socrates engaged fellow intellectual Athenians in dialectical discussions, where ideas are tested and refuted by taking opposing views. Unfortunately, he upset so many of the Athenian politicians and generals by asking too many questions of the moral and ethical structure of his society that he was tried for treason and executed.

The Socratic Method suggests that by asking open questions, it is possible to discover both answers and insights. In education, it has been found to be a very useful method of actively involving learners in thinking about important issues. However, as a slight word of caution, it may be worth remembering the fate of Socrates, and to prevent hostility, consider how you frame and ask your questions!

Conclusions: specific and general

In this section of the reflective cycle, you are asked to make conclusions. You may find that you can address this section best by asking the question 'What have I learnt?' This question in itself has several different layers. There may, for example, be considerations about the specific event. For example, I have learnt that our booking system is very efficient' or to more general learning, 'I have learnt something about what makes booking systems efficient' (e.g., realistic predictions of the time required per client). It is also important to recognise different types of learning, for example you could ask, what have you learnt about yourself? What new knowledge have you acquired? What do you understand more? Has your skill level increased?

Action planning

This part of Gibbs's reflective cycle is relatively straightforward. Here, you are being invited to decide, in the light of the information gathered, what you want to change and how you are going to go about doing it. In action inquiry, you may decide not to use this stage, as you do not need to include action planning to satisfy the methodology. When you are engaged in action planning, the aim is to initiate change, and so identifying who can influence a change is important. Reflective practice tends towards an individual activity. Thus, you are the person to carry out any immediate actions. If your discoveries from the reflective practice concern wider practice, you will need to be aware of the extent of your influence. While you may dream of reorganising the whole of your organisation, your sphere of influence may mean that this is likely to be a long-term project. No less challenging is the ability to make significant changes to our own ways of being, our habituated attitudes and behaviours. If, for instance, you tend to be quite an anxious person, and you want to become more relaxed, it needs to be a change that you feel is worth doing and for which you are highly motivated to achieve your goal.

Using other models of reflective practice

There are several different reflective models, and each has its relative methods. Many people find it helpful to have a structure to discipline their account. If you use a model to help you reflect, it is worth exploring with which you prefer to work. Along with Gibbs's model, the two most commonly used models in health and social care practice are those of Johns (2000) and Driscoll (2007).

Driscoll's model was developed from work by Borton (1970). Borton suggested reviewing events by asking the basic questions: What? So what? Now what? It is possible to see how closely related this is to Gibbs's six stages, and on the surface it appears as a significant simplification. However, Driscoll's model significantly expands on these initial questions with the use of prompt questions. These questions, shown in Box 9.1, are useful in themselves and can help when reflecting whether or not to use a particular model.

UK-based nurse academic, Chris Johns's model (Johns 1995) is probably more person-centred, rather than practice-centred, compared with either Gibbs's or Driscoll's model. Johns's model is based around the American nursing researcher, Barbara Carper's 'Patterns of Knowing' (Carper 1978). Uniquely, Johns's model was designed to be used with someone acting as a facilitator such as a mentor or clinical supervisor. Johns suggests that this dialogue with another person enables the learning from the experience to become shared (where appropriate) at a faster rate than when reflecting alone. Another aspect of Johns's model is that it brings into discussion the reflector's values and previous experiences. Over several years, Johns reviewed and revised his model based on his experiences of offering clinical supervision to practitioner colleagues. Box 9.2 illustrates one version of Johns's model.

Box 9.1   Driscoll's 2007 model of reflection.

What?
What was the purpose of the intervention?
Who was involved and what did they do?
What did you do?
Why did you do what you did?
So what ?
What were you thinking and feeling?
What was good and bad about the experience?
What skills were used or developed?
What were the consequences of your actions for the patient/relatives/colleagues?
What else could you have done?
Now what?
If it happened again, what would you do differently?
How can you improve your knowledge and skills?
How can you use what you learned from the experience in your future practice?
See also: Driscoll's reflective questions: http://www.supervisionandcoaching.com/.

Driscoll (2007)

Box 9.2   Structured model of reflection Adapted from Johns (2000: 51).

- Focus on a description of an experience that seems significant in some way
- What particular issues seem significant to pay attention to?
- How were others feeling and why did they feel that way?
- How was I feeling and why did I feel that way?
- What was I trying to achieve and did I respond effectively?
- What were the consequences of my actions on the patient, others and myself?
- What factors influence the way I was/am feeling, thinking and responding to this situation? (personal, organisational, professional, cultural)
- What knowledge did or might have informed me?
- To what extent did I act for the best and in tune with my values?
- How does this situation connect with previous experiences?
- Given the situation again, how might I respond differently?
- What would be the consequences of responding in new ways for the patient, others and myself?
- What factors might constrain me from responding in new ways?
- How do I feel about this experience now?
- Am I able to support myself and others better as a consequence?
- What insights have I gained?

Johns (2000)

Storyboarding and using other forms of art

To some extent, most of the models for reflective practice are reductionist in their approach. By this, we mean that they suggest that the questions posed can be answered in isolation from each other. The questions also force a particular structure, or approach to reflection. An alternative approach is to use art work. This could be freestyle painting or drawing or using collage. It has been used successfully to help people derive and express meaning and learning from events. You may not consider yourself an artist and may be put off by the idea, so a good alternative or place to start is storyboarding.

Storyboarding

Storyboarding is rather like creating a cartoon. It is a technique used in the animation and film industry and is used to create a structure and outline of the narrative of a film or cartoon. Storyboards may consist of a series of sequenced illustrations that allows the producer to visualise how a series of real or imaginary events can be presented.

Using the terms of reflective practice, the illustrations represent the 'description' of an event. Thought and speech 'bubbles' can be added to highlight significant moments and can include interpretations of what the significant 'actors' were thinking. The illustrations for storyboarding do not have to be complex; they can even be based on stick men. Often, the illustrations in the middle of a series represent turning points, or significant points in the event. It is interesting sometimes to compare the storyboards made by two different people that represent the same event. They can open our eyes to how each of us can experience the same events differently.

Storyboarding has been used in counselling and therapy, and as a method to help patients and clients describe how they live and experience their lives and the care services they encounter. It has also been used as an approach to help learners of health care work with complex issues such as 'end of life care' (Lillyman et al. 2011).

Artwork

Like music or mathematical symbols, art is an alternative to words for expression of ideas and experiences. The purpose of art is in some way to reflect the creator of the art, so art in itself should be generative of reflection. Thus, art work, of different media, can be effective as a means to stimulate and provoke reflection, analysis and insight. When using art work, the reflector creates a personal piece of art that embraces the nature of their experience. Both the act of creating the piece and discussing its meaning can generate deep insights into personal experiences and practices. Art work can be used to help explore personal dispositions and opinions. For example, you may choose to model an impression of yourself as a mentor using play dough or clay. As you produce the object, you will be considering yourself as a mentor and how to express these thoughts and feelings. The final object may not accurately represent these observations, but talking about your art work can bring to light a number of insights. Cortazzi and Roote (1975) invited staff from a dysfunctional health care department to create cartoon images to express what they believed was causing the difficulties, and as a result of their work facilitated significant insights that led to effective changes to the way people worked. Spouse (2000) used a similar approach when investigating nursing learners' experiences of learning in practice settings. Hughes (2009) also used it in relation to leadership education. All these authors describe how the act of creation provided great insights that led to the participants' reviewing their practice.

It is important when using these approaches not to get too carried away with the 'art' or its quality. The purpose of the activity is the depth of reflection and the learning it generates. An alternative is to create a collage of images that represent your experience, by using pictures from magazines and newspapers, and building your image by sticking them onto a larger sheet of paper.

Open reflection

Reflection is often seen as an act that is done in private, but this was not always so. Indeed, Johns's model was devised for reflection within a facilitated group. Working with other colleagues in an open group reflection requires courage and effective and agreed structures. Action learning circles are structured to help individuals to present and solve a problem that is important to them. The role of the group is to pose questions, rather than to solve the problem. The group normally has a facilitator whose role is to ensure that the group abides by the agreed rules.

Another model, although not necessarily recognised as a reflection and used by the medical profession is the 'grand round'. In a grand round, the presenting practitioner describes the problem and explains their actions to a group of fellow practitioners. The role of the fellow practitioners is to pose questions to the presenter. As with action learning circles, the questions are designed to encourage the presenter to think deeply about the problem and to consider alternatives. The success of the grand round and of action learning circles is that everyone learns from the problem. Sometimes, grand rounds, depending upon the personalities involved, can become adversarial, but often they generate more understanding and quite obviously encourage reflection.

The grand round has distinct similarities to what is known in nursing as 'clinical supervision. Clinical supervision may be a more formal relationship depending upon the facilitator and the participant/s. Sometimes it is a one-to-one relationship, and in other settings it is provided in group sessions, rather like an action learning circle. The aims of nursing clinical supervision are to promote and further develop professional practice. When clinical supervision is provided on a one-to-one basis, the supervisee is in a more junior position in the organisation than the supervisor but is not necessarily being line-managed by them. The model often used to support development of the supervisee is open, reflective and private between the individuals.

Role of empirical evidence in action inquiry

Earlier in this chapter, we described how reflection can be used as a method of inquiry into personal practice. Such approaches tend to focus on what we would call internally generated evidence, which is the view and evaluation of the person reflecting on the experience. However, a more rounded inquiry is likely to be generated if external sources of evidence are also gathered. In this next section, we will briefly explore some of those alternative sources of evidence and how they can be used.

Empirical data are data that are derived from observations; these observations are normally recorded in the form of numbers or words, and in terms of research they are normally data that have been collected in a systematic way, so as to reduce bias. In terms of everyday inquiry, this is not always possible. It is important to remember that action inquiry concerns practitioners exploring the nature of their practice and that the means needs to be appropriate to the ends. If you find that you are starting to discover significant areas where practice needs to be changed, it may be more relevant to undertake a small pilot study, or action research activity, before instigating a formal research programme. You can then check out whether your hunch is correct. If you then want to launch a larger study, your discoveries can be tested as to their applicability to other practice areas. Some areas of activity are governed by clinical protocols, and while it is appropriate to constantly question their applicability, changing them often involves the agreement of a wider community of practitioners. Some aspects of clinical practice are also subject to what is termed 'clinical governance'. This is a general term used to cover the processes and procedures that regulate practice procedures and the ways in which they are monitored and improved (Scally and Donaldson 1998). Changing practices covered under clinical governance is always required to be sanctioned by the appropriate regulatory mechanisms.

Sources of empirical data

Whatever your field of practice, you are likely to find a whole host of performance statistics: 'how many clients', 'how long it took to help them' and client satisfaction levels. Finding performance statistics is much harder when it comes to your specialist field and your workplace as a place of learning. With respect to data that can be useful and are concerned with mentoring and facilitating, you may find it helpful to know:

- the number of individuals that ask for you as a mentor/facilitator;
- the number of ex-learners that come back to you to share professional experiences;
- success rate of your learners in the placement, or their professional development;
- how long people stay in your workplace (sometime called turnover);
- the career trajectory of people that have worked with you (i.e., do they get promoted?);
- levels of short- and long-term sickness.

It is important to note that none of these measure directly the quality of your works as a mentor. They are just items of information that may tell you something worthy of further thought. Other measures that can be of value are those that relate to client outcomes or service performance, for example the number of complaints or the rate of injuries, such as slips, trips and falls or needle-stick injuries. Again, although these are not direct measures of you as a mentor, they often do indicate something about the overall learning environment in which you work. A good source of empirical data is your learners, who have a vested interest in working for change. You will find that there are many useful methods to gather data from your learners. The most commonly used approaches are questionnaires, interviews and focus groups. Box 9.3 provides an example of a question-naire you might wish to design.

Questionnaires tend to be designed to produce quantitative data (data that can be counted), as with example in the sample from a questionnaire above (Box 9.3), which asks the learner whether they thought their practice had developed during a period of learning. Typically, this would be measured by asking for a response according to a scale (see Box 9.3). Once responses have been gathered, they can then be analysed in more detail. Questionnaires like this can also include opportunities for written (qualitative) responses. Quantitative questionnaires can give a rapid impression of an experience and are useful when time is short. However, a significant drawback of quantitative survey questionnaires is that to be meaningful, you need to have more than 10 people responding. So, if you plan to use a questionnaire, it may take some time to gather enough data from a big enough sample of

---

Box 9.3   Excerpt from a questionnaire designed to assess the efficacy of a supervisor in helping to create a learning environment.

Please indicate the extent to which you agree with the following statements	Strongly agree	Agree	Neutral	Disagree	Strongly disagree
My workplace supervisor encourages me to take opportunities to learn					
I am able to take opportunities to learn					
It is easy to learn from my supervisor					

people to make your findings legitimate. You also need to be able to do the necessary data analysis either by hand or electronically. Data gathered through questionnaires, as with all data, should be considered with caution. Great effort needs to be put into the design of questionnaires to ensure that they are valid (Scott and Mazhindu 2005). This is because it is relatively easy to inadvertently write questions for questionnaires that are biased or are perceived differently by those completing the questionnaire than those who wrote it. The classic textbook on how to design and analyse questionnaires was written by Oppenheim (1992) and is worth reading before you start designing your own questionnaire. Quantitative questionnaires can be quite frustrating, as you tend to always start asking yourself, 'Why did people respond to this question like this?'

Another approach to obtaining information is by using interviews and focus groups. These are used to gather qualitative data, and generally offer richer data that will help to develop a greater understanding of the subject under inquiry. Interviews tend to be conducted on a one-to-one basis, while focus groups are normally of a group of perhaps no more than eight to 10 respondents and a facilitator who poses the questions and makes sure the conversation does not go off the topic. The advantage of a focus group is that you can obtain the views of a larger number of people in a short space of time. In addition, the group members will often have different perspectives that one person may not have considered worth discussing. Inevitably, being part of a group can be inhibiting, and individuals may not disclose as much within a group as they would to an individual interviewer. Sometimes, a focus group can be taken over by a few vocal individuals, and so the skill of the facilitator is paramount to the group's success. One significant drawback of qualitative methods is paradoxical: they generate an awful lot of data, and these data need to be sifted and sorted through with care and diligence. As with using quantitative research methods, it is a good idea to establish how you are going to analyse your data before you set out collecting them. Focus groups and interviews can be significantly biased by the person collecting the data. For instance, if you are interested in investigating your interactions with your learner, you may not be the best person to be the interviewer.

Purpose and data

As with most inquiries, the information and understanding that you gain depend on the questions that you ask and how you gather the data. For example, if you are investigating your area and practice in relation to how 'safe' your learners feel about asking questions, you need to consider whether or not you are going to ask the learners if they felt the environment was 'safe' or whether you are going to look for evidence of the effect of a 'safe' environment (such as learners asking questions) in relation to the questions asked. To do this, you need to consider the type of questions people might ask in a 'safe' environment; these could be questions that you would consider foolish, questions that were unusual and questions that were challenging. You might also choose to start your investigation by finding out from your learners whether they consider the environment safe and what this means to them. You can see in this example relating to 'safe environment' that we distinguish between measuring satisfaction, that is, 'Do the learners feel safe?' and measuring effect or the outcome of what learners describe as a safe environment. In

---

Box 9.4   Kirkpatrick's model to evaluate staff development.

- Reaction of mentee – what they thought and felt about the experience
- Learning gain – was there an increase in knowledge or capability?
- Behaviour – has there been a change in behaviour?
- Results – the effects on the organisation or clients

Box 9.5   Strategies to evaluate performance.

- Level 1: Feedback forms, sometimes referred to as 'happy sheets', as they tend to just indicate if the learner was satisfied with what they received. Such sheets, however, if well written and given after events, can yield much more useful information. Another technique is to interview learners for their more immediate reactions.
- Level 2: This level can be assessed using before-and-after tests and questionnaires, or by conducting interviews with those engaged in the development activities.
- Level 3: Here, the observations by others of the learners are probably most useful. Observation could include colleagues and clients. Interviews with the participants can also be useful, but remember you are looking for how they have changed and developed.
- Level 4: To measure this level, you will need to look at the organisational goals to see if your mentoring may have had an influence. Measuring the organisation's achievement of its goals may be relatively straightforward, but relating any change back to your own actions is difficult. However, if you are undertaking a group inquiry, you may be able to relate organisational change back to that group activity.

---

this example, the volume and quality of questions asked indicate the quality of the environment. Being able to generate 'rich' data from learners, with the many examples that they give, strengthens the quality of your findings and recommendations. Kirkpatrick (1959) developed a useful model to evaluate staff development. His model has four levels of evaluation, which are described in Box 9.4.

Kirkpatrick's model was designed to evaluate staff developments and events and programmes nevertheless it reminds us of the importance that when we are inquiring into our facilitation practice we need to explore the ultimate as well as the immediate effects. In general, the complexity and cost of obtaining valid data rise with each level of the model. Measuring the impact of coaching, mentoring and facilitation on the overall organisation can be very difficult, and it is difficult to attribute the outcomes back to the actions of the facilitators themselves. Some of the suggested methods for the different stages are provided in Box 9.5.

Strategies to evaluate performance

Kirkpatrick's (1959) model does have its detractors, particularly in relation to its over-focus on staff development as a tool for organisational change (Bates 2004). Purpose will also influence effort; for example, we have described earlier in this chapter approaches that would be recognisable as appropriate to more intensive research programmes. For the purpose of your own development, it may not be appropriate to deploy significant amounts of effort in data collection and ensuring that those data are completely free from bias (if that were ever possible). However, as you become more involved in this kind of investigation, you are likely to develop a greater level of understanding of your own practice.

Group approaches to action inquiry

Often, members of organisations or groups of people sharing similar interests (e.g., a community of practice members) will want to undertake inquiries of their collective practice. Group action inquiry brings people together that have a common interest to develop their professional understanding and practice. A suitably sized group is in the range of six to 12 people. Any more, and the group becomes unmanageable; any less, and the advantage of 'group perspective and skill' can become lost. Within the group, it is important that everyone has equal status and that all are equally co-researchers, co-decision-makers, co-participants and co-action-takers. Sometimes, the group will appoint a facilitator from a group member for each session; other times, an external facilitator will be used for the duration of the group's work together.

Confidentiality is an issue that needs to be discussed and agreed by group members. If individuals do not feel comfortable discussing sensitive issues and their concerns, then it is unlikely that members will participate openly and honestly, and significant learning will be lost. Sometimes, people adopt what are called 'Chatham House' or 'Ground' rules. These rules describe what information can be used and shared but also what information must not be discussed outside the meeting, such as the name or identity of individuals discussed and their affiliations.

Ways of working together

In this group, members decide on a programme of topics related to their professional practice. The aim is to empower group members to make their own choices. The group members work together to decide on its methods of reflection and, where appropriate, to take action. Working through this cycle of actions with each member framing and asking Socratic questions often leads to further inquiry and reflection. By being shared openly within the group, these processes can generate criticality, new ideas and new perspectives. The group progresses through the reflective cycle of thought and investigation until a point is reached when the group agrees that it has learnt all it can at that particular time and it is ready to plan and implement an action that it will subsequently evaluate.

The space of time between group meetings needs to be sufficient to allow research to take place, but not so long that momentum is lost. It is probably a good idea to start with more frequent meetings (weekly or fortnightly) until the group has learnt to work together and then to move to a situation where there is a longer period between meetings. An action inquiry group focused on a specific topic will typically last for a few months, depending upon the members' needs and wishes. When establishing an action inquiry group, it is worth remembering that its purpose is to generate understanding not necessarily to generate organisational change, and that it often enables group members to understand established practices better.

Role of the facilitator

Groups of people working together to explore practice often find it helpful to have a facilitator. The facilitator is there to help the members to work effectively with each other by respecting each other's contribution, to agree 'ground rules' and keep time, and thus to help the group to become cohesive. Another function is to help the group develop new avenues of understanding and exploration through modelling Socratic questioning if the members falter. This also helps to keep the group focused. Sometimes, groups will self-facilitate with members of the group each taking it in turns (at successive meetings) to lead the group.

Incident model

The use of models can sometimes help with group inquiry. This is because they give a distinct structure. The incident model is suitable for incidents, that is, one-offs or events that are relatively isolated, perhaps when a learner suddenly leaves the placement. So, the focus of such an incident will be what to inquire in the practices that led to the person leaving. We call this model the 'incident model'. It is based on Mitchell's (1983) model (see Box 9.6), which was originally devised for critical incident stress debriefing. It has five phases and is specifically designed to control the interaction between the groups of people involved. In our experience, the process needs to be facilitated and the facilitator needs to be relatively strict with the group so that they stick to the phase and take turns.

Action learning sets

Another potential model to use is that of the 'action learning set'. The purpose of this is different from the other forms of group inquiry that we have described, in that the group's learning is based on an attempt to support individuals within the group to

---

Box 9.6   Mitchell's (1983) critical incident model.

- Fact phase: Each person in the group, in turn describes the incident; in the case of a learner that leaves early, this would be a descriptive review (by each person) of the learner's supervision.
- Thought phase: Each person reviews their thoughts about the events that led to the incident. In the example we are using, the thoughts that each person had in relation to the progress and practice of the supervision and learning by the learner would probably be considered.
- Reaction phase: Here, we review the reactions each person had through the 'fact and thought' phase. It is to some extent analogous to the 'feelings' and 'analysis' phases of the Gibbs (1988) reflective cycle.
- After-effects phase: Each person in turn reviews what they have discovered and learnt though the incident and maybe how they have changed.
- Re-entry phase: This is an opportunity to answer any questions remaining and, if necessary, develop a plan for any future action or changes to practice.

Mitchell (1983)

explore their own individual issues, and these issues are normally work-focused. The idea of the action learning set is that by working through these issues as a group, the group itself learns. Action learning was originally devised in the United Kingdom by a senior manager, Revans (1980). Revans noticed that groups of expert scientists, when discussing their work, would go through stages of individually recognising their igno-rance, share their experiences and collectively reflect in order to learn. From these observations, he developed the method of action learning (Revans 1980), which is now used by a wide range of government organisations and businesses. Revans proposed that action learning is when: 'People need to be aware of their lack of relevant knowledge and be prepared to explore the area of their ignorance with suitable questions and help from other people in similar positions'.

A typical model of an action learning set is one in which a group of people (about eight) meet. They would agree a set of rules, for example with regard to confidentiality. Normally, at each meeting, one or two people bring to the group issues that are then to be discussed. The issues are not discussed in an open 'free for all'; instead, the person with the issue describes the issue; the group are then allowed to ask the 'issue holder' questions about the issue. It is important that within the process, the other participants do not jump to tell the 'issue holder' solutions. As with the Socratic method, the notion is that through the use of questions, suitable answers will be found. The next time the group meets, the issue holder reports back and reflects on what they have learnt. The group then moves on to another member's issue. Most action learning sets are facilitated, although Revans himself considered that facilitators were unnecessary and could inhibit the development of the group's own ability to develop its own ability to learn on its own.

Appreciative inquiry

Appreciative inquiry (AI) developed as a method for organisational change built upon an appreciation of the positive aspects of the organisation. It was developed in the United States largely for business organisations. Its positive philosophy is similar to that of the 'strengths based leadership' movement that sees the role of the leader to develop and recognise strengths rather than focusing on trying to continually rectify deficiencies. AI has a basic premise: that the questions we ask influence fundamentally the answers we find and that within the questions are often hidden our dispositions and attitudes. So, a question is seldom neutral, and if we are attempting to discover something about ourselves or our organisation, the bias within the question will influence what we find. AI also recognises that attempting to change something from a positive starting point tends to be easier than from a more negative one. The questions we ask tend also to direct our focus and lines of inquiry (Thatchenkery and Metzker 2006). So, if we ask, 'What is good about the organisation?', we will get a different understanding of the organisation than if we ask, 'What needs fixing?' Another way of thinking about this is to consider what your organisation or professional practice has, rather than what it is missing; in this way, you get an appreciation of your assets. When AI is used to formulate change, the basis of change is those assets, so it will ask the question, 'Given what your strengths are, what is the vision for this organisation?'

Four distinct phases of AI

In the original model of AI, there were four distinct phases:

- discovery;
- dream;
- design;
- destiny;

The most important phase is probably the first because it sets the tone. In the discovery phase, you ask your colleagues, self, learners, etc. to report in relation to positive questions about the issue concerned. You could, for example, be considering something like 'inclusive practice'. The classic question used by AI practitioners would be something like 'What gives strength to our inclusive practice?' Responses to these questions would be used to visualise what could be, and what would work well in the future.

In the design phase, participants decide what the organisation or individual will actually seek to achieve, and plans how to accomplish it. The destiny phase is when plans are implemented.

If AI is used for large-scale organisational change, then often the process starts with as many of the significant stakeholders as possible. The meeting, often called an AI summit, attempts to work through the first three phases of the AI process. The aim of the summit is to gain maximum support and to engender a positive attitude towards the organisation.

The AI process has had significant success and is now widely used by management consultants. The process is used by the National Support Teams, which form part of the United Kingdom's National Health Service. It has also been used as part of change processes by universities in the United Kingdom (Cousins 2008).

Summary

Action inquiry is a powerful approach to investigating, understanding and developing both professional practice and organisational functioning. Action inquiry assumes that even the everyday is worthy of exploration. Action inquiry combines multiple methods of inquiry, such as reflection alone or in different types of groups. It can include collecting empirical data and is aimed at facilitating and generating change through the people who are most closely involved in everyday activities.

Chapter 10

Personal and professional development planning

Ian Scott

Introduction

This chapter will explore how you can undertake a range of professional development activities that will enhance your skills as a mentor and facilitator. It will examine how to set goals and develop planned activities so that you can meet these goals. The chapter also discusses what to look for when choosing a mentor/facilitator for yourself.

This chapter includes the following:

- an outline of professional development;
- goal setting;
- finding a vision;
- the role of values;
- planning your development;
- recording achievement.

Personal and professional development planning

In some ways, this book has been entirely about professional and personal development, but it has concerned you as a facilitator of someone else's professional development. In Chapter 9, we looked at ways of inquiring into your practice as a facilitator, which is an excellent departure point for considering your own professional development.

Personal and professional development has always taken place, although in recent years there has been an increase in expectations and opportunities. Across all the professions, documentary evidence of personal professional development has become a standard requirement. Alongside this growth in professional development and its recording has been an emphasis on professional and personal development planning, often termed PDP. Within the United Kingdom, for instance, Higher Education institutes (HEIs) are now required to provide ongoing personal development planning to students, the idea being that students exit their programmes with a portfolio of evidence of their achievements.

Practice-Based Learning in Nursing, Health and Social Care: Mentorship, Facilitation and Supervision,
First Edition. Ian Scott and Jenny Spouse.
© 2013 John Wiley & Sons, Ltd. Published 2013 by John Wiley & Sons, Ltd.

Defining professional development

Professional development can be defined as the act of engaging in activities that maintain and enhance your capabilities as a professional.

You will recognise that within this definition is an assumption that if you do not engage in professional development, your capabilities as a professional are likely to decrease. This of course is largely because health and social care are fast-moving fields, where if you do not keep up with contemporary practices and beliefs, you get left behind. Inevitably, there is always a potential for complacency to creep into personal practice. This has inevitable consequences for personal satisfaction and client safety. Certainly, in terms of university teachers, Marsh (1987) has produced compelling evidence that without formal professional development, satisfaction ratings for individual teachers tend to drift downwards overtime. The range of activities that constitute professional development are potentially very wide. These activities can embrace both informal development activities such as serious discussions in journal clubs or case conferences with colleagues and more formal activities such as following an educational programme, online or at an AEI.

Recording professional development (and achievement) has more recently become an important element of PDP. Within UK Higher Education, PDP was given great impetus by the influential Dearing report (NCIHE 1997), which investigated the provision of adult education in the United Kingdom. The introduction of PDP was seen originally by its proponents as a way of promoting liberal education values and student-centred learning (Jackson 2001). The Quality Assurance Agency (QAA) guidelines define PDP as: 'a structured and supported process undertaken by a learner, to reflect upon their own learning, performance and achievement, and to plan their educational and career development' (QAA 2009: 5). Obviously, these guidelines are written with a view to learners throughout the adult education system rather than for their educators. There exists within the literature some debate as to whether PDP is for the self, as an individual within the world and generated by personal self-generated goals and aspirations, that is, whether its focus is purely personal or professional development. This difference is important because it influences the purpose of the process. In addition, a personal plan is likely to be a private enterprise, while a professional development plan could be influenced by a range of interested parties.

Most health and social care professionals will have a requirement to undertake continuing professional development, to record it and to have those records available for scrutiny by their professional body. So, our emphasis in this chapter is on professional development planning, although inevitably personal growth will also take place.

Professional development planning and appraisal systems

It is easy to confuse appraisal systems used by organisation personnel departments and PDP. This is because human resources and personnel departments have changed over the years to become much more focused on human-resource development (see Marchington and Wilkinson 2008). There is also a superficial similarity in the structure PDP processes and some of those processes used in appraisal. If we look at these two approaches in more detail, we can see there is a significant difference in their philosophy, process and purpose.

Differences in purpose

Appraisal

The purpose of appraisal is to enhance the capability of an organisation and to make judgements about an individual's performance. From the appraisal, individual goals are set, and needs are established in relation to those goals.

PDP

PDP, on the other hand, is overtly concerned with your development as a professional. The goals are those set for yourself, guided by your professional needs. PDP seeks to help you to plan how you meet those goals and how to record your learning on the journey to meet them.

In the next section, we will look at goal setting as the basis for PDP. You will probably recognise that much of the discussion and the approaches we shall be exploring can also be used with anyone you are facilitating.

Goal setting

Goal setting is probably one of the hardest aspects of PDP. Goals can be tangible and easy to measure, such as 'to become higher paid' or 'to acquire a specific new skill'. They can also be more nebulous and harder to know when they have been achieved, for example 'giving better feedback'.

Unlike appraisal systems, being able to measure the achievement of a goal is not that important in PDP. It is of far greater importance that the goal setting leads to purposeful developmental activity, learning and reflection. A goal is not necessarily a target; it should be seen as a general direction of travel. Goals should be achievable, and you need to describe how you will be satisfied that you have reached each particular goal.

Timescales

Timescales are worth considering when setting goals. Some goals may be achievable very rapidly, while others may take much longer. If your goal is to become a representative of your professional statutory regulatory organisation (PSRO) or any other of your profession's organisations, such as its ruling council, it may take longer to achieve than if your goal is to learn how to teach a particular skill to a group of students. Longer-term goals obviously take longer to achieve. A PDP that is only made up of long-term goals can generate despondency. Achieving your goals is important for your motivation and thus your commitment. When developing your PDP, we recommend that you have a mix of long-, medium- and short-term goals. Sometimes, longer-term goals will require their own separate plan. Activities that lead to the overall goal are termed objectives. Objectives tend to be more easily measurable, but this is not necessarily so.

As this book has been written for a range of different professionals, it is difficult for us to provide examples of specific goals. We have nevertheless provided a few ideas (Box 10.1).

Box 10.1   A variety of short- and long-term goals for a typical workplace mentor/ facilitator.

Short-term goals
I will assess my learner's capability and document it before delegating any activities
I will always discuss a shift work plan with my learner and agree priorities and actions, which I will check mid-shift and at the end of the shift
I will look at ways in which I can improve documentation of my learners' progress
I will develop my network of contacts across the organisation

Long-term goals
I will take and complete a short (6-month) course in an area related to my specialist practice
I will become more involved in the decision-making processes in my organisation
I will negotiate to become an assessor in the skills lab at the AEI

Determining your goals can be difficult, and sometimes it is hard enough to think about maintaining things as they are, rather than constantly trying to develop and change. As a health or social care practitioner, you are working in an environment where there are constant technological developments influencing practice, and where changes in legislation and public attitudes influence working practices and resources. Intellectually and professionally, standing still is no longer an option! By actively planning and setting your own goals, you will be taking control of your own destiny. Having said this, determining your own goals can still be challenging for some people.

Finding a vision of you

A technique that can help in goal setting is known as 'back-casting'. Back-casting is a technique that was originally used by planners of large-scale developers and was first described being used in development planning by Scott et al. (2010–2011). Back-casting is an envisioning technique used to develop pathways to goal attainment. The technique is built on working back from a significant 'destiny' goal (Drebourg 1996).

Back-casting

Back-casting is an envisioning technique that encourages you to see where you could be or where you want to be. Without such a goal, it is often difficult to develop and sometimes to escape the routine of daily existence.

Begin this activity by sitting somewhere quietly. Imagine, for example, that you are employed in your perfect professional working environment. Now, focus on what you think someone whom you might admire in that environment is doing. Perhaps it is the leader or someone who is particularly adept and accomplished. Now, consider *how* these people are functioning and what skills and attributes they have. Imagine now that you are seeking to develop similar capabilities; consider what skills and attributes you would need a stage in your career, before gaining this capability. As you work backwards, you will discover a career path built by developing positive attributes, skills and knowledge. These skills and attributes of your ideal person are just one step away from where you are now, and you can use them to formulate your goals.

Other visioning techniques

Treasure trove

An alternative visioning technique to back-casting is to imagine that you have just discovered a hidden treasure trove. Inside that trove are all the professional attributes, knowledge and skills that you have ever wanted. All you need to do is to describe what is there. Give yourself a minute to write down what you want to take from the box. Now, for each attribute or skill, ask yourself 'Why do I want that item?'

If you can produce a convincing argument, then such an attribute, aspect of knowledge or skill should be incorporated into your professional goals.

Newspaper article

Imagine that you are reading a newspaper article about your professional career, written about you 10 years in the future. What would that article say? What are the achievements that it describes?

This is a much harder exercise than it sounds, so you may want to ask two trusted friends to write this type of article for you. Often our friends have better (or at least different) insights into our true abilities and, perhaps, desires than we do.

Appreciative inquiry

Appreciative inquiry (AI) is a technique that we described in Chapter 9. It is normally used in the context of formulating a vision for an organisation, but you can also adapt it for yourself or your learner.

AI is a four-stage process. In the first stage, you gather positive comments about yourself, for example about you as a mentor, as a practitioner or as a manager. These could be gathered from immediate colleagues, managers and your students, and it is important that your informants understand that AI only works with the positive. The principle behind AI is that it is better to build a vision on the positives. The second stage is about producing a vision.

Using the AI approach, you can use the information gathered in stage 1 to build a picture of your potential, what you could be. While, for most people, embarking on AI seems a scary idea, experience suggests that it is invariably an uplifting and rewarding experience.

Using art

In Chapter 9, we suggested ways in which using images (collages) or creating images of any kind can help to elicit pre-conscious knowledge. Hughes (2009) and others have developed ways of using art in the coaching and mentoring process. A significant aspect of this process is to help learners to establish their own vision and hence goals. You can use any kind of art form, but Hughes's work suggests that it tends to be either sculpture or some form of drawing/painting. If you would like to use art, you may want to try drawing an image of yourself as a professional a few years in the future.

If you are not a visual person, you may find using sounds (birdsong, music and so on) as a means of describing how you want to be in the future. Constructing the image is a valuable way of thinking about yourself and your aspirations, and the image that you produce is a memory tag, or souvenir. It can serve as an anvil for conversations about your goals, but you can also keep it as reminder of your aspirations.

Using probing questions

The visioning techniques described above tend to rely on our ability to create an image of ourselves in the future with relative ease. For some people, this is a tricky process, as they may not think in images of sound or shape. They may be unsure of their aspirations for themselves as a professional. An alternative approach is to use a series of probing questions that attempt to discover their aspirations. Table 10.1 provides a list of questions that you might like to use. It is not exhaustive. You could use a Likert scale to score your responses on a 1–5 scale (5 highest, 1 lowest), for the level of agreement with the statement. As with all the techniques, being honest with yourself is important.

Table 10.1   Sample questions.

Question	Strongly agree 5	Agree 4	Neither 3	Disagree 2	Strongly disagree 1
I always feel good when I am working with patients/clients					
I always feel good when talking with patient/clients					
Working with learners is a positive experience for me					
I enjoy taking the lead					
I prefer communicating in writing					
I enjoy giving presentations					
I enjoy organising people					
I feel good when I am in charge					
I always feel good taking responsibility for others					
I enjoy organising teams					
I like working across a range of organisations					
I would like to be top management					
I am good at making decisions					
I enjoy supervising others					
Public speaking is easy for me					
The esteem of others is important to me					
I enjoy routine work					
The clinical work situations I enjoy most are…? Why do I enjoy them?					

Table 10.2 How important are these values to you?

Value	Importance to you	Value	Importance to you
Possessions		Capability	
People		Caring	
Love		Surviving	
Loyalty		Fairness	
Freedom		Sacrifice	
Dedication		Integrity	
Ambition		Tolerance	
Education		Money	

Importance of values

Sometimes we do not set appropriate goals for ourselves because we do not recognise our own values and desires. This is why it is so important to consider your vision of yourself in the future, before you set your goals. If you find it difficult to create a vision, a good alternative is to have a strong idea of your own values.

Values are concepts that you consider significant in the way you live. They tend to determine your true priorities and have a strong influence on your actions and behaviours. When your actions are in accord with your values, you tend to be happy. If there is a mismatch between your actions and beliefs, the dissonance is likely to lead to unhappiness. Look at the values listed in Table 10.2, and score the terms of how important they are to you. Are there any other values that you can add to the list? Do they represent your values? Do they represent the values shown within your workplace?

Our values tend not to change throughout our lives; they are linked to our cultural background and our education, and there is some evidence that they have a genetic component. Often, we find that people with similar careers have similar values. Sometimes, organisations have similar values, even though on the surface they might not be expected to. For example, the values of the United States Army are: loyalty, duty, respect, selfless service, integrity and personal courage. To what extent do these values accord with yours or those of your organisation? Why do you think this may be?

Where are you now?

A good next step is to undertake an honest review, working out your current skills and strengths. As with most aspects of professional planning, this is often harder than it seems because our ability to accurately estimate our own prowess varies. In Chapter 1, we listed a range of attributes and skills required of facilitators of learning. If you do some research, you can probably find a similar list for other career paths. With such a list, it is possible to score yourself and gain some appreciation of your own 'skill' set. An alternative, and probably more reliable, approach would be to ask your colleagues and mangers to do the scoring, if you feel you can trust them to be honest and sincere. But this anticipates the kind of working relationship you and your colleagues enjoy within your workplace.

An alternative approach to identifying your existing skills and attributes is to remember times and periods from your life, both within and outside work, when you were successful. This could be something as (seemingly) simple as organising a successful children's party to performing a complex series of clinical procedures. Using memories like this, you can record those factors and the things that you did that made you successful. If you use a wide range of experiences, you are likely to gain a good understanding of your skills and attributes.

Goal setting

Hopefully, you have now got a better sense of where you want to go, and the skills and attributes that you want to develop. So, now you need to translate these into goals. There are several models available to help with this, the most well known being the SMART model, although strictly speaking the SMART model is normally applied to the setting of objectives. SMART stands for:

- specific – in that they apply to a particular activity with a well-defined end result;
- measurable – you will know when the goal is achieved;
- achievable – the goal can be achieved and is not nebulous;
- realistic – the goal is attainable;
- time-based, having a specific end-date achievement.

Remembering the list of goals we described earlier in this chapter (Box 10.1), most of them comply to this model. For example, the goal, 'I will assess my learner's capability and document it before delegating any activities' seems to fit quite well; you will certainly know when it is achieved; it is specific and measurable; and it includes a time limit. Whether it is realistic and achievable will depend on how well you organise your time when you are supervising a learner.

There are of course some critical positions on the SMART approach, notably that it does not support goals that are less easy to measure, such as 'I will become more involved in the decision-making processes in my organisation' (see Box 10.1). The fact that SMART assigns a time to complete a goal can create anxiety. Life has a way of intervening in long-term plans, so be flexible. The downside of SMART is that the demand for a goal to be realistic and achievable can lead to formulating simplistic and easily reached goals.

The SMART approach evolved from the work of Locke and Latham (1990). If you take a quick look at their original work, it shows the extent to which the notion of setting SMART goals has over-simplified Locke and Latham's original principles. These principles were that goal setting needs to reflect:

- clarity;
- challenge;
- commitment;
- feedback;
- task complexity.

The SMART planning model (rather than Locke and Latham's 1990 model) also seems to deny the need for commitment from the originator. They argue that you have to really want to achieve the goal; otherwise it probably will not happen.

So, goal setting is more complex than is suggested by the SMART model, and when setting your own goals you need to ask yourself questions such as: 'Do I really want to achieve this goal?', 'Does this goal fit with my personality and beliefs?', 'Is this goal challenging?' and 'Will I know if I am progressing towards achieving the goal?'

In working through these aspects, do not be afraid to acknowledge your true motivation. You may be striving to improve yourself so that you can do your best for your learners, but factors such as prestige and earning more money could be as important to you.

Do not forget to record your goals. When you write down your goals and record them, you are more likely to regard them as imported when compared with those that you do not record.

Points to ponder:

- Is the following statement a reasonable goal, and does it fit with the models described? 'I will become a very effective mentor'
- How could it be adapted to match the SMART model?
- Do you think the statement should it be adapted, and if you do, why?

Tactics when setting goals

There are a few things to aim to achieve when setting your goals; these include the following:

- make your goals explicit and realistic;
- ensure your goals do really reflect who you are and what you want;
- use a realistic time frame;
- make sure your goals are meaningful and worthwhile, but not so challenging that they cannot be achieved;
- recognise and develop the skills and knowledge that you need to achieve each goal;
- recognise that your self-esteem is different and separate from achieving your goals (a difficult challenge).

Professional recognition as a clinical educator

As a facilitator of learning in the workplace, it may be that one of your goals is to gain professional recognition for this meaningful and worthwhile activity. Across professions and national boarders, requirements for recognition, or indeed whether or not recognition is available, vary. With the development of understanding of how people learn has come recognition of the importance of the workplace facilitator to the professions and a skill that needs to be fostered and developed. With this understanding comes recognition of the importance of appropriate professional qualifications and specific preparation for people who take responsibility for developing others.

Some professions have structured routes and programmes that lead to formal recognition of the role. In the United Kingdom, examples of these are found in requirements of the professional statutory regulatory organisations, such as the Nursing and Midwifery

Council and the Health and Care Professions Council for the United Kingdom. The PSROs of these professions have articulated the knowledge skills and understanding required by those that educate, and particularly those that assess their novices. To become a formally recognised mentor or supervisor, in health or social care practice, requires successful completion of a post-qualification course, approved by the relevant professional body. This textbook has covered the requirements of such PSROs.

Becoming a mentor, facilitator or supervisor

For nurses in the United Kingdom, a four-stage process is currently recognised (Nursing and Midwifery Council of the United Kingdom 2008a, b) as follows:

Stage 1: professional registration

This stage is achieved on registration with the Nursing and Midwifery Council following successful completion of an approved programme. Within the standards of pre-registration nursing, midwifery and health visiting, it is recognised that mentors or clinical supervisors should be able to '. . . facilitate students and others to develop their competence' (Nursing and Midwifery Council of the United Kingdom 2008a, b).

Stage 2: mentor

Individuals that achieve Stage 2 of the standards are known as 'mentors'. These individuals have direct responsibility for facilitating the learning of a specific learner or group of learners. The mentors are expected:

- to have the knowledge and skills to build effective relationships in order to facilitate learning;
- to provide appropriate learning opportunities;
- to develop effective learning environments;
- to assess students.

Stage 3: practice teacher

Practice teachers are responsible for organising and co-ordinating learning activities of pre-registration students. Such individuals tend to have the responsibility of a group of students and be responsible for supervising a team of mentors, although in health visiting education, mentors are known as practice teachers

Stage 4: teacher

A teacher is someone who organises and facilitates learning both in practice and in classroom situations within an AEI. Typically, they may also be known as a lecturer. In the United Kingdom, those who reach Stage 4 must also demonstrate that they meet the professional standards described in the descriptor for the United Kingdom professional standards for teaching in Higher Education (HEA 2011). In general, those who teach health professionals in university settings possess a professional qualification, a higher degree (either a Masters or a doctorate) and a teaching qualification. It is normal for those new to tutoring in higher education to gain their teaching qualification during the first two years of their first teaching post (Source: Nursing and Midwifery Council of the United Kingdom 2008a, b).

The requirements of the NMC can be contrasted with that for medical educators in the United Kingdom. Currently, while the general medical council (GMC) does require that senior clinicians have the skills to facilitate learning, there is no requirement for those responsible for the education of doctors to hold a post-registration a teaching qualification.

If you have as a long-term goal a career in facilitating learning in clinical practice, you need to understand the requirements of your PSRO and to set your goals accordingly.

Priority setting

Following goal setting, the next step in professional development planning is priority setting. Priority setting combines three inter-related concepts: importance, immediacy and order.

Importance

Importance refers to how important this particular goal is to you. Importance may be determined by a range of factors and will almost certainly relate to your own personal motivation, but could also be driven by the demands of your workplace organisation. You may, for example, want to devote time to your goal to become a practice teacher. On the other hand, your practice area manager may need you to master a particular clinical skill so that you can teach it others. Agreeing to a short-term goal may help you with your long-term goals. So, complying with your manager's request may well help you to persuade them to give you time at a later date to complete a course to become a mentor or a practice teacher. Thus, it is easy to see how a goal that was not originally yours can assume more importance for you than the real goal you are aiming at. It also illustrates how a changing external environment can influence the priority we place on our goals.

Being honest with yourself has a significant bearing on achieving your goals, if you consistently do not manage to find the time to complete a goal; it is probably because that goal, in reality, is not that important to you. It is of course possible to be swamped by other people's goals (such as in the example above). So, being able to set effective and realistic goals of your own can help. It is also worth remembering the relationship between goals and values that we described above. If you consistently find that you miss your goals, you may find it useful to seek help from your own trusted mentor or someone who understands your work, either inside or outside your organisation, who you can use as a personal coach.

One obvious method to help prioritise is to list your goals and then score them according to importance. Table 10.3 shows a set of priorities for a hypothetical midwife mentor called Amber.

Table 10.3   Amber's goals and their importance to her professional development.

Goal	Importance scale 1–6 (6 = most important)
Enable my next allocation of students to thrive on placement to the best of their abilities	5
Become more confident in documenting my decisions after assessing my learner(s)	3
Learn how to undertake perineal suturing (for my manager)	1
Give a presentation to colleagues on how to select an appropriate catheter size (for my manager)	1
Become a practice teacher	1
Undertake and successfully complete a practice teacher course	2
Improve the quality of my documentation	4

In Table 10.3, you can see that Amber has made the requests from her manager to complete training in perineal suturing and giving a talk to her colleagues, top priorities. She is clearly hoping that this may help her with her other goals. Note also that Amber's importance scoring may not be the same as yours. Why might this be?

Immediacy

Some goals need to be attended to with more urgency than others. If we look at Table 10.3, we can see that Amber has decided that she needs to help the team learn more about the correct choice of catheter. We can presume that this decision has been made because of the need to update both herself and her colleagues. It is probable that she was asked to give this session because of a related incident or issue, and the manager is hoping to avoid a recurrence or a more serious clinical incident to occur. This indicates that goals have professional importance as well as personal importance. It is possible to have situations where a neglected goal can suddenly assume a much greater level of importance than it would otherwise.

The immediacy with which a goal needs to be completed thus has an impact on its priority. So, we could add a new column to Box 10.1 to indicate which goals need to be completed in the short term and which could wait a while. We can see from Table 10.4 that Amber now has a goal 'Give a presentation to team on how to select an appropriate catheter size', which, although it has an importance score (to Amber) of 1, has an immediacy of 6 and thus would leap to the top of her list of priorities. Of course, these 'immediacy' scores are contestable, and you may disagree with Amber; perhaps her manager would, too.

The last aspect of priority setting is to deal with order; put simply, some goals must come before others. In Amber's example (Table 10.4), we know that Amber must complete a practice teacher course successfully before she can become one. It is also probable, although not essential, that Amber will want to improve her documentation and the quality of her assessment decisions before undertaking her practice teacher course.

Table 10.4   Amber's goals and their importance to her and their immediacy.

Goal	Importance	Immediacy
	1 = low, 6 = high	
Enable my next allocation of students to thrive on placement to the best of their abilities	5	5
Become more confident in documenting my decisions after assessing my learner(s)	3	4
Learn how to undertake perineal suturing (for my manager)	1	6
Give a presentation to colleagues on how to select an appropriate catheter size (for my manager)	1	6
Become a practice teacher	6	1
Undertake and successfully complete a practice teacher course	6	2
Improve the quality of my documentation	4	3

Challenging the barriers

So, you have decided on your vision and set some goals for yourself. What next? Some writers would suggest that you should take each goal and set objectives around them. Objectives being measurable, sub-divisions of goals. In my mind, however, this very much depends on how broadly you have set your goals. If your goal is to become prime minister, setting objectives is probably a good step. If your goals are already quite specific, then setting further objectives may simply be an exercise in potentially using lots of paper and creating unnecessary work. One thing that is worth while doing, however, is assessing whether there are any barriers (actual or potential) to achieving your goals and how you could go about removing or ameliorating the barriers. Barriers can be either perceived or real. You need to consider both types.

Some of the most common barriers to individual professional development are associated with personal factors:

- lack of motivation;
- lack of time;
- lack of management support;
- lack of direction;
- lack of finance;
- too many goals;
- fear of failure;
- lack of realism;
- a chaotic lifestyle;
- lack of ability;
- not having goals.

From this list, you can see that the most common reasons are often inter-linked. For instance, if you are leading a rather chaotic lifestyle and as a consequence not getting sufficient sleep, then, even though your desire may be strong, it is highly unlikely that you will be motivated sufficiently to succeed. Many barriers can be overcome. You will be

Table 10.5 Potential barriers to achieving goals and approaches to tackling them.

Barrier	Tackling the barrier
Lack of motivation	Try a detailed re-examination of your goals Look at your lifestyle Examine your commitments Consider what you will gain if you successfully reach your goals List your successes, skills and positive attributes Try setting yourself just a few, achievable short-term goals
Lack of time	Making more time is probably impossible, so if you are struggling to reach a goal you must re-organise your commitments. This may mean having serious conversations with your manager, or even seeking a post that can leave time for commitment to your goals.
Lack of management support	The best way to gain management support is to align your goals to those of your manager. Find out how their performance is being measured, and rationalise the way you present your goals to them in the light of this. So, what are your manager's priorities and can you align yours with them? It is probably worth considering alternative ways to develop yourself, not all of which require management support, for example volunteering.
lack of direction	Spend some time trying to locate your vision for yourself. Try setting just a few short-term goals.
lack of finance	Formal professional training tends to be paid for either by the employer or by the employee. If you can demonstrate why your goals will benefit your employer, you are more likely to get their financial support. Banks will often provide loans for professional training, and charities supporting professional education will also provide funding if you make a satisfactory case.
Too many goals	Set priorities for your goals, and do not add to the list until some are completed
Fear of failure	Professional education rarely fails to produce professional development. You have very little to lose.
Lack of realism/ability	If you are setting goals that are too challenging, you may never reach them. Focus your efforts on areas where you have evidence that you have strengths.
Not having goals	You know the answer to this one! Relocate your vision, and find some goals for your professional life.

aware of this if you think about some of the circumstances and achievements of your patients and clients. Table 10.5 gives a few approaches that you can use to address such a range of potential barriers.

Recording your goals

The process described above requires a reasonable amount of effort; however, your investment will pay off. Research is conclusive that those individuals who set specific goals for themselves tend to be more successful than those who do not. Making a formal record of your goals helps you to emphasise your commitment. Recording your goals also helps with a review process. The more public your commitment to your goals, the greater effort you are likely to invest in trying to achieve them. Some people will want to keep their goals private; this is perfectly reasonable, and there are many reasons for this. We would recommend, however, that you record your goals in a place where you can see them easily. After all, your goals should be an important aspect of your life! There are a range of formats that you can use to record your goals. We shall be discussing some approaches to recording your goals later in this chapter.

Professional development opportunities

There is an immense range of activities that you can undertake to help with your professional development. By reading this book, you have become familiar with a range of approaches to stimulate professional learning and these apply to you as much as to the learners you are working with.

In general, learning opportunities can fall into two categories (described in Chapter 1): planned and unplanned. Planned opportunities can be further divided into formal structured activities and those that have structure but are less formal. Often, when people talk about continuing professional development, they tend to put great importance on formal structured learning, even though by far the greatest amount of CPD takes place informally.

Formal structured activities

Formal structured opportunities for professional development tend to be provided by in-house training departments, independent trainers, whose services are paid for by the employer, and Adult Education Institutions (AEIs). You can use formal opportunities to develop practical skills (such as resuscitation skills), as well as to extend your knowledge, understanding and social network.

Employers often provide a range of mandatory courses (e.g., fire safety, moving and handling patients) as well as a wide portfolio of additional courses. This often depends on the size of organisation and their staff training and development budget. The course may extend over a number of days, although more often they are short half- or one-day courses, so as to minimise the disruption to staffing levels. Courses provided by an employer seldom include formal assessments of what has been learnt, although they may evaluate the processes.

Opportunities provided by AEIs tend to take place over a wider time frame (often a number of months or even years) and the learning tends to be provided in discrete modules of related material, which are formally assessed. Modules are offered at different academic levels. Successful completion of an accredited module or course leads to the award of academic credit. Academic credit is rather like currency in that it can often be used towards a specific award, at a particular academic level, such as an honours degree or Master' degree. Once a certain amount of credit has been accumulated, if the value of the credit matches the requirements of a degree programme a full degree may be awarded. Often, credit can be transferred across AEIs and even between countries (particularly within the European Union). Unfortunately, not all AEIs use the same credit system. If you want to apply for a degree using credits that you have already gained, you need to check that the AEI will recognise and accredit them toward the degree you want to do.

Increasingly formal structured professional development opportunities are being provided online or are provided face to face but have a component of the support available online. Most AEIs expect learners to be computer-literate and that you will have access to a computer. In general, the skills needed to access learning opportunities provided online are similar to those used for electronic documentation of records in your workplace, or for social networking and online shopping.

Online learning has many advantages. You do not have to attend classes at a certain time, you can study when you want to, learning materials and activities tend to be readily available, and you do not need to spend time and money travelling into classes. However, they can be expensive.

The downside of online learning can be that people feel they are studying in isolation and that the level of interaction is less. Providers of online education often address this problem by having chat rooms, or social-media sites, so there are opportunities for live discussion. Sometimes, people are more willing to express their anxieties and weaknesses when they are online than when face to face. As technology and software to support this type of activity develop, so such opportunities are improving. Skype, using a computer with a microphone and video, is a good way to be part of a synchronous online conference call.

Online courses and attendance-based courses (at an AEI) both have similar success rates (passing assessments). Course completion rates tend to favour face-to-face teaching. An important point to remember about online learning is that it takes as much time as face-to-face learning. Online learning provides more choice as to when and where you study. If you do not have enough time to complete a face-to-face course, it is unlikely that you will have enough time for an online course either, so it is worth working through your existing commitments and what you can drop in order to free up the necessary time, before you opt for one or other type of course.

Less formal and informal activities

Most purposeful learning tends to fall under this heading. As we discussed in Chapter 9, informal workplace learning can include activities such as job shadowing, action learning sets, case reviews, discussions with a mentor/facilitator, action inquiry in all its forms and undertaking research. Activities such as learning from a book or the Internet can be just as beneficial. Indeed, there is now so much information available on the Internet, it might be considered that the role of formal learning opportunities is diminishing. For example, if Amber were to conduct a search of the Internet for videos on suturing techniques, she will find several hundred available; the trick of course is to determine their quality.

For all the activities described above, we know that they are made more powerful when the activities are planned and supported by considered reflection on what has been learnt. It is probably true that anything that can be learnt in a formal setting can probably also be learnt through the less formal route just as well. Taking one of Amber's goals, 'Give a presentation to team on how to select an appropriate catheter size' (Table 10.4), it may be that in order to do this, Amber will want to brush-up on her presentation skills. She can decide whether she should go on a formal course or maybe watch a few of the many training videos available through the Internet and do a practice presentation in front of her mentor.

Amber may recognise that the less formal approach is much cheaper than the formal route, but does she have the confidence? Will she actually be able to dedicate her time to this activity, or would she find it easier to devote time by attending formal classes? Amber may find that if she attends and successfully completes a formal course, she will be able to record this on her curriculum vitae (CV), and perhaps use the credits towards an honours degree or a post-graduate certificate, depending on the education provider.

Opportunistic and accidental learning experiences

Opportunistic and accidental learning experiences are those that are completely unplanned. This is probably the most common form of learning. It occurs throughout our lives and should not be forgotten when considering our professional development. Opportunistic and accidental learning often occurs most, when we take part in new experiences or experience an event that has never happened to us before. It can of course also occur when we hear something new from the television or radio. Using processes such as reflection or journal keeping (see Chapter 9) can help us to harvest and consolidate learning from such experiences. Not only will these processes help you learn, but because you have had to think about how and what to document, you are more likely to be able to talk about your experiences. This can be very helpful when you are involved in selection processes such as a job interviews.

Reviewing and reflecting

As you undertake professional development activities, be they informal or formal, it is a good idea to take some time out to review what you have learnt and how far it has taken you towards your goals. Any of the models described in Chapter 9 are suitable for this activity. Try to make a record of what you feel you have learnt, go beyond what you intended and ask yourself hard questions such as:

- As a result of this course, how have I changed my behaviours?
- As a result of this course, in what ways have my skills developed?
- What changes have my colleagues noticed?
- In what way has this development activity changed outcomes for my patients/clients/students?

As part of the review process, do not be afraid to reconsider and, if necessary, rewrite your goals. Do you still consider them to be achievable? Are you on track to complete them? How would you score progress so far? Are your goals still sufficiently challenging? Are there any goals that you feel you will now really struggle to complete, and if so, can you identify what the significant barriers are? Are your direction and vision still the same?

Recording your achievements

Recording your achievements is a significant aspect of professional development planning. The act of recording is empowering and brings motivation. Recording can be part of a document or series of documents that incorporates your goals and reflections on your learning and development. Such a series of documents is sometimes called a portfolio, although quite often a portfolio is just a place where practitioners (including health professionals) store evidence of their work and their achievements (certificates) they have throughout their career.

Whatever we shall call it, the importance of these documents is not the documents but the process through which the document is brought together. This is normally the kinds of activities that we have described in Chapter 9 and in this chapter. We would recommend that you use the same document for your goals, reviewing, reflections and achievements. Such documents do not need to be bulky; indeed, we recommend making and storing your documents in electronic format and, if necessary, maintaining a separate file for your certificates (not forgetting to back them up, in case your computer dies). Using digital storage allows documents to be more dynamic, and you can use different forms of media, such as your art work, music, poetry, photographs and voice recordings.

When making these documents, remember that their real purpose is to support your learning and to help you when it comes to describing your professional self to others. By this, we are encouraging you to choose a format for your documents that works best for you, because they are not for public consumption. We would recommend that you use these two headings:

• my vision;
• my goals.

When writing each goal, describe what you are going to do, and how, in order to achieve it. For each goal, have a section devoted to reflecting on your progress and what you have gained by undertaking the activities. Lastly, have a section entitled achievements, where you record: your successes, both past and present, and your achievements, experience, attributes and skills.

AEIs often provide their students with an online environment to use to maintain their records of achievement and to build their portfolio. These have a similar structure to those that we have described in this chapter. The United Kingdom National Health Service also provides access to a bespoke e-portfolio system for its staff. Most of these software systems give you an advanced approach to storing and filing information in a manner that makes it easy to collect. Some software systems include prompts to go through reflective cycles, and some also help you to build web-based commentaries about your experiences. There are, however, some issues with such online systems; for example:

• they require you to learn a new piece of software;
• they are often too complex for some people;
• they have functionality that most people do not need;
• they often lack transferability between systems.

For many people, it is just as easy to store the information using standard word-processing-based software.

The danger with using digital media is its vulnerability to loss and damage. However, now that storage is easily and freely available online (cloud technology), this is much less of an issue, and of course if you really want to, there is always paper.

Closing the circle: finding your own mentor/facilitator

We hope that by now, you can recognise the value and importance of a mentor/facilitator to develop professionals and that in planning your own development, we hope you will consider finding such a person.

From the research on workplace facilitators and mentors, it is clear that they function at their best when there exists a good working relationship between learner and facilitator. Inevitably, it is more satisfactory when the 'learner' can choose their facilitator. Other than formal training and education programmes, you are free to make this choice. The person that you choose does not need to come from your workplace. Indeed, many freelance professional coaches are employed by organisations, precisely because they bring an external view that allows employees to see beyond the immediate context of their work environment. The question, of course, is what to look for in your mentor/facilitator. Here are a few questions that you can ask yourself that may help you to decide.

Questions to use when choosing a mentor/facilitator

First, ask yourself, 'What are the three most important qualities (be specific) that I am looking for in my mentor?' Having identified these qualities, then ask, 'Does this person have similar values to me?' If the answer is 'No' to this question, move on in your search. A good mentoring relationship depends on people having similar values. The third significant question to ask is, 'What do I want from my mentor?' (again be specific).

Once you have established the answers to these questions, you can then move on to more 'domestic issues'; good questions to ask yourself here are:

- Will I be able to form an effective professional relationship with this person? Do I respect them?
- Does this person have the knowledge, networks and skills that are important to me?
- Does this person have time for me? Are they available?
- Does this person want to mentor me?
- Will this person be sufficiently challenging?
- Is this a person who will be able to find out who I am and what drives me?

Be professional and systematic about how you choose a mentor. Make a list of potential people and systematically go through that list asking yourself the type of questions that are described above about each person. Do not be afraid to interview a potential mentor; tell them that you are interested in potentially using them as your mentor and that you would like to discuss this with them. People are invariably flattered by such approaches, and of course, it is good for their CV as well. Do not be afraid to decide that a particular person you have contacted is not right for you; after all it is your life and your career. Do remember that you are allowed to have more than one mentor.

There are some people who you may want to avoid as mentors, even though they meet your requirements. For instance, avoiding anyone with immediate line-management responsibility for you is probably a good idea, as is anyone with whom you have had a close relationship. It is also wise to avoid those individuals who have dominant characters who may want to 'tell you' what to do. After all, you will learn best by discovering for yourself.

If a mentoring relationship is not going well for you, end the relationship; there is no point in carrying on with something that is not helping you. A mentoring relationship should be primarily about you and your professional development needs. End the relationship in a professional way by explaining to your mentor why you have to move on. A good mentor will understand your reasons and would have learnt from their own experiences with you.

Summary

Professional development planning is a process that can help individuals to develop their careers and strengthen their practice. Planned development is often more effective than that which is ad hoc. Setting goals and working towards these goals gives focus, brings motivation and helps us to recognise our own successes. Because of social and professional changes, there is a wide variety of both formal and informal development opportunities available to health and social care professionals. By using these techniques of review and reflection, you can make your own mentoring and facilitation skills stronger and so support your learners to achieve their potential.

References

Alexander, M.F. (1982) Integrating theory and practice in nursing. *Nursing Times Occasional Papers*, 17 & 18, 65–71.

Argyris, C. (1982) *Reasoning, Learning and Action: Individual and Organisational*. Jossey Bass Publishers, San Francisco.

Atherton J.S. (2011) *Teaching and Learning; What Works and What Doesn't*. www.learningand teaching.info/teaching/what_works.htm

Atkins, S. & Williams, A. (1995) Registered nurses experiences of mentoring undergraduate nursing students. *Journal of Advanced Nursing*, 21, 1006–1015.

Bates, R. (2004) A critical analysis of evaluation practice: the Kirkpatrick model and the principle of beneficence. *Evaluation and Program Planning*, 27, 341–347.

Beard, C.M. & Wilson J. (2002) *The Power of Experiential Learning*. Kogan Page, London.

Beard, C.M. & Wilson, J. (2006) *Experiential Learning: A Best Practice Handbook for Educators and Trainers*, 2nd edn. Kogan Page, London.

Belenky, M.F., Clinchy, B.M., Goldberger, N.R. & Tarule, J.M. (1986) *Women's Ways of Knowing: The Development of Self, Voice and Mind*. Basic Books, New York.

Benner, P. (1982) From novice to expert. *American Journal of Nursing*, 82, 402–407.

Benner, P. (1984) *From Novice to Expert; Excellence and Power in Clinical Nursing Practice*. Addison-Wesley, Menlo Park, CA.

Benner, P., Tanner, C.A. & Chesla, C.A. (eds) (1996) *Expertise in Nursing Practice: Caring Clinical Judgement and Ethics*. Springer, Cambridge, MA.

Berthold, J.S. (1968) Symposium on theory development in nursing. Prologue. *Nursing Research*, 17, 196–203.

Biggs, J.B. (1996) Enhancing teaching through constructive alignment. *Higher Education*, 32, 347–364.

Birch, J. (1975) *To Nurse or Not to Nurse: An Investigation into the Cause of Withdrawal During Nurse Training* . Royal College of Nursing of the United Kingdom, London.

Bjørk, I.T. (1999) Practical skill development in new nurses. *Nursing Inquiry*, 6, 34–37.

Borton, T. (1970) *Reach, Touch and Teach*. Hutchinson, London.

Boud, D., Keogh, R. & Walker, D. (1985) *Reflection: Turning Experience into Learning*. Kogan Page, London.

Boud, D., Keogh, R. & Walker, D. (1996) Promoting reflection in learning. In: *Boundaries of Adult Learning* (eds R. Edwards, A. Hanson & P. Raggart). Open University Press, London.

Practice-Based Learning in Nursing, Health and Social Care: Mentorship, Facilitation and Supervision, First Edition. Ian Scott and Jenny Spouse.
© 2013 John Wiley & Sons, Ltd. Published 2013 by John Wiley & Sons, Ltd.

Bourdieu, P. (1991) *Language and Symbolic Power* (ed. J.B. Thompson, transl. G. Raymond & M. Adamson). Polity Press, Oxford.

Bowlby, J. (1988) *A Secure Base: Clinical Application of Attachment Theory*. Routledge, London.

Bradby, M. (1990) Status passage into nursing: Another view of the process of socialisation into nursing. *Journal of Advanced Nursing*, 15, 1220–1225.

Brim, O.G. & Wheeler, S. (1966) *Socialization After Childhood: Two Essays*. John Wiley, New York.

British Dyslexia Association (2012) Website. www.bdadyslexia.org.uk

Brunner, J. (1987) Life as narrative. *Social Research*, 54, 11–32.

Buber, M. (1937) *I and Thou*. Edinburgh, T and T Clark. Translated by Ronald Gregor Smith, English translation, 2nd (revised) edn 1958.

Campbell, A.V. (1984) *Moderated Love*. SPCK, London.

Campbell, D., Jones, S. & Brindle, D. (2008) 50 injuries, 60 visits—failures that led to the death of Baby P. *The Guardian* (London). www.guardian.co.uk/society/2008/nov/12/baby-p-child-protection-haringey

Carper, B. (1975) *Fundamental patterns of knowing*. Unpublished PhD thesis, New York Teacher's College, Columbia University.

Carper, B. (1978) Fundamental patterns of knowing in nursing. *Advances in Nursing Science*, 1, 13–23.

Carr, W. & Kemmis, S. (1986) *Becoming Critical: Education, Knowledge and Action Research*. Falmer Press, London.

Chittenden, E.H., Henry, D., Saxena, V., Loeser, H. & O'Sullivan, P.S. (2009) Transitional clerkship: an experimental course based on workplace learning theory. *Academic Medicine*, 84, 872–876.

City and Guilds (2005) *Level 2 in NVQ in Health (3173)*. City and Guilds, London.

Cortazzi, J. & Roote, S. (1975) *Illuminative Incident Analysis*. McGraw Hill, London.

Cousins, G. (2008) Researching learning. In: *Higher Education: An Introduction to Contemporary Methods and Approaches*. Taylor & Francis, Abingdon, UK.

Cox, A. (2005) What are communities of practice? A comparative review of four seminal works. *Journal of Information Science*, 31, 527–540.

Coy, M.W. (1989) *Apprenticeship: From Theory to Method and Back Again*. State University of New York Press, Albany, NY.

Damasio, A.R. (1999) *The Feeling of What Happens: Body, Emotion and the Making of Consciousness*. Vintage, London.

Darling, L.A.W. (1984) What do nurses want in a mentor? *Journal of Nursing Administration*, 14, 42–44.

Darling, L.A.W. (1985) The mentoring dimension: Can a non-bonder be an effective mentor? *Journal of Nursing Administration*, February, 30–31.

Davies, A. (2000) *Effective assessment in art and design: writing learning outcomes and assessment criteria in art and design*. Project Report. CLTAD, University of the Arts, London.

Davis, F. (1975) Professional socialization as a subjective experience. The process of doctrinal conversion among student nurses. In: *Sociology of Medical Practice* (eds C. Cox. & A. Mead), Chapter 6, pp. 116–131. Macmillan, Collier, London.

Day, R.A., Field, P.A., Campbell, I.E. & Rutter, L. (1995) Students evolving beliefs about nursing: from entry to graduation in a four year baccalaureate programme. *Nurse Education Today*, 15, 356–364.

Deci, E.L. & Ryan, R.M. (1985) *Intrinsic Motivation and Self Determination in Human Behaviour*. Plenum, New York.

Dewey, J. (1939) *Experience and Education*. Collier Books/Macmillan, New York.

Dodd, P. (1973) Toward an understanding of nursing. Unpublished PhD thesis, University of London.

Drebourg, K. (1996) Essence of backcasting. *Futures*, 28, 813–828.

Dreyfus, H.L., Dreyfus, S.E. & Benner, P. (2009) Implications of the phenomenology of expertise for teaching and everyday comportment. In: *Expertise in Nursing Practice: Caring, Clinical Judgement and Ethics* (eds P. Benner, C.A. Tanner & C.A. Chesla), Chapter 10, 258–280. Springer, New York.

Dreyfus, H.L. & Dreyfus, S.E. (1986) *Mind over Machine: The Power of Human Intuition and Expertise in the Era of the Computer.* Basil Blackwell, Oxford.

Driscoll, J. (2007) *Practising Clinical Supervision: A Reflective Approach for Healthcare Professionals.* 2nd ed. Bailliere Tindall Elsevier, Edinburgh.

Duffy, K. (2003) *Failing Students: A Qualitative Investigation of Factors That Influence the Assessment of Students' Competence to Practice.* Glasgow Caledonian University. www.nmc-uk. org/Documents/Archived%20Publications/1Research%20papers/Kathleen_Duffy_Failing_Students2003.pdf

Eby, L. (1997) Alternative forms of mentoring in changing organizational environments: a conceptual extension of the mentoring literature *Journal of Vocational Behaviour*, 51, 125–144.

Edmond, C.B. (2001) A new paradigm for nursing practice education. *Nurse Education Today*, 21, 251–259.

Eraut, M. (1985) Knowledge creation and knowledge use in professional contexts. *Studies in Higher Education*, 10, 117–133.

Eraut, M. (2003) The many meanings of theory and practice. *Learning in Health and Social Care*, 2, 61–65.

Eraut, M. (2010) *Balance Between Communities and Personal Agency: Transferring and Integrating Knowledge and Know-How Between Different Communities and Contexts.* learningtobe professional.pbworks.com/f/michael+eraut+D3.pdf

European Union (2005) Directive 2005/36/EC of the European Parliament and of the Council of 7 September 2005 on the recognition of professional qualifications. *Official Journal of the European Union*, L255, 22–142.

Fretwell, J. (1982) *Ward Teaching and Learning: Sister and the Learning Environment.* Royal College of Nursing, London.

Fretwell, J. (1985) *Freedom to Change: The Creation of a Ward Learning Environment.* Royal College of Nursing, London.

Fuhrer, U. (1993) Behaviour setting analysis of situated learning. In: *Understanding Practice: Perspectives on Activity and Context* (eds S. Chaiklin & J. Lave), pp. 171–211. Cambridge University Press, Cambridge.

Gibbs G. (1988) *Learning by Doing: A Guide to Teaching and Learning Methods.* Oxford Further Education Unit, Oxford Polytechnic, Oxford.

Gibbs, G. & Simpson, C. (2004–2005) Conditions under which assessment supports students' learning. *Learning and Teaching in Higher Education*, 1, 3–31.

Goody, E.N. (1989) Learning, apprenticeship and the division of labour. In: *Apprenticeship: From Theory to Method and Back Again* (ed. M.W. Coy), pp. 233–256. State University of New York Press, Albany, NY.

Gott, M. (1984) *Learning Nursing: a Study of the Effectiveness and Relevance of Teaching Provided During Student Nurse Introductory Course.* Royal College of Nursing of the United Kingdom, London.

Graves, B. (1989) Informal aspects of apprenticeship in selected American occupations. In: *Apprenticeship: From Theory to Method and Back Again* (ed. M.W. Coy), pp. 51–64. State University of New York Press, Albany, NY.

Gray, M.A. & Smith, L.N. (2000) The qualities of an effective mentor from the student nurse's perspective: Findings from a longitudinal qualitative study. *Journal of Advanced Nursing*, 32, 1542–1549.

Haas, J. (1989) The process of apprenticeship: ritual, ordeal and the adoption of the cloak of competence. In: *Apprenticeship: From Theory to Method and Back Again* (ed. M.W. Coy), pp. 87–114. State University of New York Press, Albany, NY.

Habermas, J. (1984) *Theory of Communicative Action. Volume 1: Reason and the Rationalization of Society*. Translated by: T. McCarthy. Polity Press/Blackwell, Cambridge.

Hamilton Smith, S. (1972) *Nil by Mouth?* Royal College of Nursing of the United Kingdom, London.

Hart, G. & Rotem, A. (1994) The best and worst experiences: students experiences of clinical education. *The Australian Journal of Advanced Nursing*, 11, 26–33.

Hattie, J. (2009) *Visible Learning: A Synthesis of Over 800 Meta-Analyses Relating to Achievement*. Routledge/Taylor & Francis, London.

Hattie, J. & Timperley, K. (2007) The power of feedback. *Review of Educational Research*, 77, 81–112.

Hauer, K.E., Holmboe, E.S. & Kogan, J.R. (2011) Twelve tips for implementing tools for direct observation of medical trainees' clinical skills during patient encounters. *Medical Teacher*, 33, 27–33.

Hay, J. (1995) *Transformational Mentoring*. McGrawHill Book Company, New York.

HEA (2011) *The UK Professional Standards Framework for Teaching and Supporting Learning in Higher Education*. http://www.heacademy.ac.uk/assets/documents/ukpsf/ukpsf.pdf

Health & Safety Executive (2012) Website. www.hse.gov.uk/disability/

Hempstead, N. (1988) *Nursing Recruitment, Retention and the Nursing Environment: A Survey of Views of Third Year Nurses in the Oxford Region*. Oxford Regional Health Authority, Oxford.

Henderson, A., Cooke, M., Creedy, D.K. & Walker, R. (2011) Nursing students' perceptions of learning in practice environments: a review. *Nurse Education Today*, 32, 299–302.

Heron, J. (1981) Philosophical basis for a new paradigm. In: *Human Inquiry: A Source Book for New Paradigm Research* (eds P. Reason & J. Rowan), Chapter 2, 19–35. John Wiley, Chichester, UK.

Hill, F. (2007) Feedback to enhance student learning: Facilitating interactive feedback on clinical skills. *International Journal of Clinical Skills*, 1, 21–4.

HM Government (2010) *Disability & Equality Act*.

Hochshild, A.R. (2003) *The Managed Heart: Commercialisation of Human Feelings (20th Anniversary Edition 2003)*. University of California Press, Berkley, CA.

House, V. (1977) Attitudes to degree course and shortened course for graduates: Interviews with ward sisters/ charge nurses. *Nursing Times Occasional Paper*, 31 March, 41–44.

Hughes, S. (2009) Leadership, management and sculpture: how arts based activities can transform learning and deepen understanding. *Journal of Reflective Practice*, Special Issue 10.1.

Illeris, K. (ed.) (2009) *Contemporary Theories of Learning*. Routledge, London.

Isles, P. & Freer, R. (1999) Students helping students. *Kai Tiaki Nursing New Zealand*, June 18–19.

Jacka, K. & Lewin, D. (1989) *The Clinical Learning of Student Nurses*. NERU Report No. 6. King's College University of London, London.

Jackson, N. (2001) Personal development planning: what does it mean? The Higher Education Academy. www.heacademy.ac.uk/…/id465_pdp_what_does_%20it_%20mean.pdf

James, D. (2005) Importance and impotence? Learning outcomes and research in further education. *The Curriculum Journal*, 16, 83–96.

Jang, H. (2008) Supporting students' motivation, engagement, and learning during an uninteresting activity. *Journal of Educational Psychology*, 100, 798.

Jarvis, P. (2009) Learning to be a person in society: Learning to be me. In: *Contemporary Theories of Learning* (ed. K. Illeris). Routledge, London.

Johns, C. (1995) Framing learning through reflection within Carper's fundamental ways of knowing in nursing. *Journal of Advanced Nursing*, 22, 226–34.

Johns, C. (2000) *Becoming a Reflective Practitioner*. Blackwell Publishing, Oxford.

Jones, A. (2010) Attachment, belonging and identity are important in health curricula. *Nurse Education Today*, 30, 277–278.

Jones, D.C. (1974) *Food for Thought*. Royal College of Nursing of the United Kingdom, London.

Jordan, B. (1989) Cosmopolitical obstetrics: Some insights from the training of traditional midwives. *Social Science and Medicine*, 28, 925–944.

Jourard, S.M. (1971) The 'manners' of helpers and healers. The bedside manners of nurses. In: *The Transparent Self* (ed. S.M. Jourard), pp. 179–207. Van Nostrand Reinhold, New York.

Kegan, R. (1982) *The Evolving Self: Problems and Processes in Human Development*. Harvard University Press, Cambridge, MA.

Kilminster, S., Zukas, M., Quinton, N. & Roberts, T. (2010) Learning practice? Exploring the links between transitions and medical performance. *Journal of Health Organization and Management*, 24, 566–570.

Kilminster, S., Zukas, M., Quinton, N. & Roberts, T. (2011) Preparedness is not enough: understanding transitions as critically intensive learning periods. *Medical Education*, 45, 1006–1015.

Kirkpatrick, D.L. (1959) Techniques for evaluating training programs. *Journal of ASTD*, 11, 1–13.

Kluger, A.V. & DeNisi, A. (1996) The effects of feedback interventions on performance: A historical review, a meta-analysis, and a preliminary feedback intervention theory. *Psychological Bulletin*, 119, 252–284.

Knight, P. & Yorke, M. (2003) *Assessment, Learning and Employability*. SRHE/Open University Press, Maidenhead, UK.

Kogan, J.R., Holmboe, E.S. & Hauer, K.E. (2009) Tools for direct observation and assessment of clinical skills of medical trainees: a systematic review. *Journal of the American Medical Association*, 302, 1316–1326.

Kram, K.E. (1985) *Mentoring at Work: Developmental Relationships in Organizational Life*. Scott, Foresman, Glenview, IL.

Lamond, N. (1974) *Becoming a Nurse: The Registered Nurses' View of General Student Nurse Education*. Royal College of Nursing and National Council of Nurses of the United Kingdom, London.

Lave, J. & Wenger, E. (1991) *Situated Learning: Legitimate Peripheral Participation*. Cambridge University Press, Cambridge.

Levett-Jones, T. & Lathlean, J. (2008) Belongingness: A pre-requisite for nursing students' clinical learning. *Nurse Education in Practice*, 8, 103–111.

Levett-Jones, T., Lathlean, J., McGuire, J. & McMillan, M. (2007) Belongingness: A critique and implications for nursing education. *Nurse Education Today*, 27, 210–218.

Lewin, K. (1948) *Resolving Social Conflicts; Selected Papers on Group Dynamics*. G. W. Lewin (ed.). Harper & Row, New York.

Lewis, M.A. (2006) Nurse bullying: organizational considerations in the maintenance and preparation of health care bullying cultures. *Journal of Nursing Management*, 14, 52–58.

Lillyman, S., Gutteridge, R. & Berridge, P. (2011) Using a storyboarding technique in the classroom to address end of life experiences in practice and engage student nurses in deeper reflection. *Nurse Education in Practice*, 11, 179–185.

Locke, E. & Latham, G.P. (1990) *A Theory of Goal Setting & Task Performance*. Prentice Hall, New York.

Longley, M., Shaw, C. & Dolan, G. (2007) *Nursing Towards 2015. Alternative Scenarios for Health Care, Nursing and Nurse Education in the UK 2015*. Nursing and Midwifery Council. www.nmc-uk.org

Luker, K. (1984) Reading nursing: The burden of being different. *International Journal of Nursing Studies*, 21, 1–7.

MacGuire, J.M. (1970) Attrition from nursing training. *International Nursing Review*, 17, 135–141.

Mackay, L. (1989) *Nursing a Problem*. Open University Press, Milton Keynes.

Maggs, C.J. (1983)*The Origins of General Nursing*. Croom Helm, London.

Manthey, M. (1980) *The Practice of Primary Nursing*. Blackwell Scientific, Boston.

Marchington, M. & Wilkinson, A. (2008) *Human Resource Management at Work: People Management and Development*. CIPD, London.

Marsh, H.W. (1987) Students' evaluations of university teaching: research findings, methodological issues, and directions for future research. *International Journal of Educational Research*, 1 (3) (entire issue).

Marsick, V.J. (1987) *Learning in the Workplace*. Croom Helm, London.

Marton, F. & Säljö, R. (1976a) On qualitative differences in learning: I outcome & process. *British Journal of Educational Psychology*, 46, 4–11.

Marton, F. & Säljö, R. (1976b) On qualitative differences in learning: II outcome as a function of the learner's conception of the task. *British Journal of Educational Psychology*, 46, 115–127.

Maslow, A. (1954) *Motivation and Personality*. Harper & Row, New York.

Maslow, A. (1970) *Toward a Psychology of Being*, 2nd edn. Van Nostrand Reinhold, New York.

May, N., Veitch, L., McIntosh, J.B. & Alexander, M.F. (1997) *Preparation for Practice: Evaluation of Nurse and Midwife Education in Scotland, 1992 Programmes*. Glasgow Caledonian University. Funded by National Board for Nursing, Midwifery and Health Visiting for Scotland.

McDougall, M. & Beattie, R.S. (1997) Peer mentoring at work: the nature and outcomes of non-hierarchical developmental relationships. *Management Learning*, 28, 423–437.

McKimm, J., Jollie, C. & Hatter, M. (2007) Mentoring theory and practice. Developed from 'Preparedness to practice, mentoring scheme' July 1999. NHSE/Imperial College School of Medicine.

Mead, G.H. (1934) *Mind, Self and Society*. Chicago University Press, Chicago.

Melia, K. (1981) *Student nurses' accounts of their work and training: a qualitative analysis*. Unpublished PhD thesis, University of Edinburgh.

Melia, K.M. (1987) *Learning and Working: The Occupational Socialisation of Nurses*. Tavistock Press, London.

Menzies, I.E.P. (1970) *The Functioning of Social Systems As a Defence Against Anxiety*. The Tavistock Institute of Human Relations, London.

Mezirow, J. & Associates (2000) *Learning as Transformation: Critical Perspectives on a Theory in Progress*. Jossey-Bass, San Francisco.

Mitchell, J.T. (1983) When disaster strikes. The Critical Incident Stress Debriefing. *Journal of Emergency Medical Services*, 8, 36–39.

Mogan, L. & Knox, J. (1987) Characteristics of best and worst clinical teachers as perceived by university faculty and students. *Journal of Advanced Nursing*, 12, 331–337.

NCIHE (1997) *Higher Education in the Learning Society*. HMSO, Norwich, UK.

NHS (2012) Dyslexia. www.nhs.uk/choices

NHS Choices (2012) www.nhs.uk/nhsengland/nsf/pages/mentalhealth.aspx

Nicholson, N. (1987) Work, role transitions: progress and outcomes. In: *Psychology at Work* (ed. P. Warr), pp. 160–177. Penguin Books, Harmondsworth, UK.

Nicol, J.M., Bavin, C.J. & Fox, H.A. (1996) Assessment of clinical and communication skills: Operationalizing Benner's model. *Nurse Education Today*, 16, 175–179.

Nolan, C.A. (1998) Learning on clinical placement: the experiences of six Australian student nurses. *Nurse Education Today*, 18, 622–629.

Nuffield Provincial Hospitals' Trust (1953) *The Work of Nurses in Hospital Wards: a Report of a Job Analysis*. Oxford Provincial Hospitals Trust, Oxford.

Nursing and Midwifery Council of the United Kingdom (2008a) *Standards to Support Learning and Assessment in Practice*. Nursing and Midwifery Council of the United Kingdom, London. Publication 01/07/2008.

Nursing and Midwifery Council (2008b) *Standards of Conduct, Performance and Ethics for Nurses and Midwives*. Nursing and Midwifery Council of the United Kingdom, London. www.nmc-uk.org/Nurses-and-midwives/Standards-and-guidance1/The-code/The-code-in-full/

Nursing and Midwifery Council (2009) *Record Keeping: Guidance for Nurses and Midwives*. Nursing and Midwifery Council of the United Kingdom, London. www.nmc-uk.org/Documents/Guidance/nmcGuidanceRecordKeepingGuidanceforNursesandMidwives.pdf - 2010-05-19

Nursing and Midwifery Council (2010a) *Guidance for Raising and Escalating Concerns*. Nursing and Midwifery Council of the United Kingdom, London. www.nmc-uk.org/.../Past-consultations/By-year/Guidance-for-raising-and-escalating-concerns/

Nursing and Midwifery Council (2010b) *Standards of Proficiency for Pre-Registration Nursing Education*. Nursing and Midwifery Council of the United Kingdom, London. www.nmc-uk.org

Nursing and Midwifery Council UK (2011) *NMC UK Wide Quality Assurance Framework, Mott Macdonald Audit Trail of Assessment of Programme Approval Requirements: Pre-Registration Nursing 2012*. www.nmc.mottmac.com/infoprogproviders/

Nursing and Midwifery Council of the United Kingdom (2012) *NMC UK Wide Quality Assurance Framework, Mott Macdonald Audit Trail of Assessment of Programme Approval Requirements: Pre-Registration Nursing 2012*. www.nmc.mottmac.com/infoprogproviders/

Ogilvie, S. (2004) Guilds, efficiency, and social capital: evidence from German proto-industry. *Economic History Review*, 57, 286–333.

Oppenheim, A.N. (1992) *Questionnaire, Design, Interviewing and Attitude Measurement*. London, Continuum Press.

Ormrod, J.E. (1999). *Human Learning*, 3rd edn. Upper Saddle River, NJ: Prentice-Hall.

Owen Hutchinson, J. & Atkinson, K. (2010) *Into Physiotherapy: Welcoming and Supporting Disabled Learners*, The Chartered Society of Physiotherapists, downloaded, 2012.

Parker, P. (2009) What should we assess in practice? *Journal of Nursing Management*, 17, 559–569.

Parkes, K.R. (1985) Stressful episodes reported by first-year student nurses. A descriptive account. *Social Science Medicine*, 20, 945–953.

Pawson, R. (2004) *Mentoring Relationships: An Explanatory Review*. ESRC UK Centre for Evidence Based Policy and Practice: Working Paper 21.

Pearson, J. (1978) *Educational Encounters in the Ward*. Unpublished MPhil thesis, CNAA, Polytechnic of North London.

Pendleton, D., Scofield, T., Tate, P. & Havelock, P. (1984) *The Consultation: An Approach to Learning and Teaching*. Oxford University Press, Oxford, pp. 347–364.

Piaget, J. (1972) Intellectual evolution from adolescence to adulthood. *Human Development*, 15, 1–12.

Polanyi, M. (1966) *The Tacit Dimension*. London, Doubleday.

Powell, D. (1982) *Learning to Relate? A Study of Student Psychiatric Nurses' Views and Their Preparation and Training*. Royal College of Nursing of the United Kingdom, London.

Quality Assurance Agency (2003) *Learning from Subject Review 1993–2001*. QAA, Gloucester.

Quinn, F. (1995) *The Principles and Practice of Nurse Education*, 3rd edn. Stanley Thornes Publishers Ltd, Cheltenham, UK.

Reid, N.G. (1985) *Wards in Chancery: Nurse Training in the Clinical Area*. Royal College of Nursing of the United Kingdom, London.

Revans, R. (1980) *Action Learning: New Techniques for Management*. Blond & Briggs, London.

Rogers, C. (1961) *On Becoming a Person: A Therapist's View of Psychotherapy*. Constable, London.

Rogers, C. (1969) *Freedom to Learn: A View of What Education Might Become*, 1st edn. Merill, Columbus, OH.

Rogers, C. (1983) *Freedom to Learn in the 80's*. Merill, New York.

Rowntree, D. (1977) *Assessing Students: How Shall We Know Them?* Harper & Row, London.

Ryan, R.M. & Deci, E. (2000) Self determination theory and the facilitation of intrinsic motivation, social development and well-being. *American Psychologist*, 55, 68–78.

Scally, G. & Donaldson, L.J. (1998) Clinical governance and the drive for quality improvement in the new NHS in England. *British Medical Journal*, 317, 61–65.

Schön, D. (1983) *The Reflective Practitioner*. Jossey Bass, San Francisco.

Schutz, A. (1970) *On Phenomenology and Social Relations: Selected Writings* (ed. H.R. Wagner). University of Chicago Press, Chicago.

Scott, G.A. (2004) *Does Socrates have a Method?* Pennsylvania State University Press, Pennsylvania.

Scott, I. & Mazhindu, D. (2005) *Statistics for Health Care Professionals: An Introduction*. Sage, London.

Scott, I. (2011) The learning outcome in higher education: time to think again? *Worcester Journal of Learning and Teaching*. 5. www.worc.ac.uk/adpu/1124.htm

Scott, I., Takavarasha, C. & Thompson, S. (2010–2011) Developing leaders through work-based learning, back-casting and partnership. *Learning and Teaching in Higher Education*, 4, 146–149.

Seed, A. (1995) Crossing the boundaries – experiences of neophyte nurses. *Journal of Advanced Nursing*, 21, 1136–1243.

Silverman, J.D., Kurtz, S.M. & Draper, J. (1996) The Calgary–Cambridge approach to communication skills teaching. Agenda-led, outcome-based analysis of the consultation. *Education in General Practice*, 7, 288–299.

Simpson, I.H. (1967) Patterns of socialisation into the professions. The case of student nurses. *Sociological Inquiry*, 37, 47–54.

Singleton, J. (1989) Japanese folk craft pottery. In: *Apprenticeship: From Theory to Method and Back Again* (ed. M.W. Coy), pp. 13–30. State University of New York Press, Albany, NY.

Skinner, B.F. (1953) *Science and Human Behaviour*. Macmillan, New York.

Smith, P. & Gray, B. (2001) Re-assessing the concept of emotional labour in student nurse education. *Nurse Education Today*, 21, 230–237.

Smith, P. & Lorentzon, M. (2008) The emotional labour of nursing. In: *Common Foundation Studies in Nursing* (eds J. Spouse, M. Cook & C. Cox), 4th edn, Chapter 3, pp. 67–88. Churchill Livingstone, Edinburgh.

Smith, P. (1992) *The Emotional Labour of Nursing*. Macmillan, Basingstoke.

Spouse, J. (1990) *An Ethos for Learning*. Scutari Press, London.

Spouse, J. (1996) The effective mentor: A model for student learning in clinical practice. *Nursing Times Research*, 1, 120–133.

Spouse, J. (1998) *Understanding learning in the professional context: 6 case studies of nursing learners*. Unpublished PhD thesis, University of Bath.

Spouse, J. (2000) An impossible dream? Images of nursing held by pre-registration learners and their effect on sustaining motivation to become nurses. *Journal of Advanced Nursing* 32 (3), 730–739.

Spouse, J. (2001) Bridging theory and practice in the supervisory relationship: a socio-cultural perspective. *Journal of Advanced Nursing*, 33, 512–522.

Spouse, J. (2003a) Learning to be a professional. In: *Professional Learning in Nursing*. Blackwell Science, Oxford, Chapter 6, pp. 158–184.

Spouse, J. (2003b) *Professional Learning in Nursing*. Blackwell Science, Oxford.

Stobart, G. (2006) The validity of formative assessment. In: *Assessment and Learning* (ed. J. Gardner). Sage, London.

Taylor, M. (1987) Self directed learning: More than meets the observer's eye. In: *Adult Learning from the learner's perspective* (eds D. Boud & V. Griffin), Chapter 14, pp. 179–196. Kogan Page, London.

Thatchenkery, T. & Metzker, C. (2006) *Appreciative Intelligence: Seeing the Mighty Oak in the Acorn*. Berrett-Koehler Publishers, San Francisco.

The Lord Laming (2009) *The Protection of Children in England: A Progress Report*. The Stationery Office, London. Retrieved 12 March 2009.

The Quality Assurance Agency for Higher Education (2009) *Personal Development Planning: Guidance for Institutional Policy and Practice in Higher Education*. www.qaa. ac.uk/academicinfrastructure/progressfiles/guidelines/pdp/pdpguide.pdf

Thomas, S.P. & Burk, R. (2009) Junior nursing students' experiences of vertical violence during clinical rotations. *Nursing Outlook*, 57, 226–231.

Torbert, W. (2010) The practice of action inquiry. In: *Handbook of Action Research: The Concise Paperback Edition* (eds P. Reason & H. Bradbury). Sage, London.

Vallint, S. & Neville, S. (2006) The relationship between student nurse and nurse clinician: impact on student learning. *Nursing Praxis in New Zealand*, 22, 23–33.

Vygotsky, L. (1978) *Mind in Society: The Development of Higher Psychological Processes* (eds M. Cole, V. John-Steiner, S. Scribner & E. Souberman). Harvard University Press, Cambridge, MA.

Watson, J. (2009) Caring science and human caring theory: Transforming personal and professional practices of nursing and health care. *Journal of Health & Human Services Administration*, 31, 466–482.

Wenger, E. (1998) *Communities of Practice: Learning, Meaning and Identity*. Harvard University Press, Cambridge, MA.

Wertsch, J. (1991) *Voices of the Mind: A Sociocultural Approach to Mediated Action*. Harvester Wheatsheaf, London.

Whaite, I. (2003) Professional standards and rules. In: *Common Foundation Studies in Nursing* (eds J. Spouse, M. Cook & C. Cox), Chapter 4, pp. 89–124. Churchill Livingstone, Edinburgh.

Wilson-Barnett, J., Butterworth, T., White, E.M., Twinn, S., Davies, S. & Riley, L. (1995) Clinical support and the Project 2000 nursing student: factors influencing this process. *Journal of Advanced Nursing*, 21, 1152–1158.

Wisdom, H. (2012) *Mentor's experiences of supporting pre-registration nursing students. A grounded theory study*. Unpublished EdD thesis, The Open University.

Wood, D. (1998) *How Children Think and Learn*, 2nd edn. Blackwell, Oxford.

Wood, D., Bruner, J. & Ross, G. (1976) The role of tutoring in problem solving. *Journal of Child Psychology*, 17, 89–100.

Wright, L.R. (1975) *Bowel Function in Hospital Patients*. Royal College of Nursing of the United Kingdom, London.

Wyatt, J.F. (1978) Sociological perspectives on socialisation into a profession: A study of student nurses and their definition of learning. *British Journal of Educational Studies*, 26, 263–276.

Yates, P., Cunningham, J., Moyle, W. & Wolin, J. (1997) Peer mentorship in clinical education: outcome for first year learners. *Nurse Education Today*, 17, 508–514.

Yorke, M. (2011) Assessing the complexity of professional achievement. In: *Learning to Be Professional Through a Higher Education* (ed. N. Jackson), e-book. learningtobeprofessional. pbworks.com/w/page/15914947/FrontPage

Zohar, D. (1990) *The Quantum Self*. Bloomsbury Publishing, London.

Index